# Short Essay Questions
# for
# MRCOG Part 2

# Short Essay Questions for MRCOG Part 2
## A self-assessment guide

**Pallavi Latthe** MD MRCOG
Specialist Registrar, Obstetrics and Gynaecology

**Khalid S. Khan** MBBS FCPS MSc MRCOG MMEd
Consultant Obstetrician and Gynaecologist and
Honorary Senior Lecturer, Obstetrics and Gynaecology

**Janesh K. Gupta** MBChB MSc MD MRCOG
Clinical Senior Lecturer and Honorary Consultant,
Obstetrics and Gynaecology

**Harold Gee** MD FRCOG
Consultant Obstetrician and
Honorary Senior Lecturer, Obstetrics and Gynaecology,
Director of Postgraduate Medical Education,
Director of Part 2 MRCOG Course

*Department of Obstetrics and Gynaecology,
Birmingham Women's Hospital,
Birmingham, UK*

A member of the Hodder Headline Group
LONDON

First published in Great Britain in 2001 by Arnold,
a member of the Hodder Headline Group
338 Euston Road, London NW1 3BH

http://www.arnoldpublishers.com

Co-published in the United States of America by
Oxford University Press Inc.
198 Madison Avenue, New York, NY10016
Oxford is a registered trademark of Oxford University Press

Whilst the advice and information in this book are believed to be true and
accurate at the date of going to press, neither the authors nor the publisher
can accept any legal responsibility or liability for any errors or omissions
that may be made. In particular (but without limiting the generality of the
preceding disclaimer) every effort has been made to check drug dosages;
however it is still possible that errors have been missed. Furthermore,
dosage schedules are constantly being revised and new side-effects
recognized. For these reasons the reader is strongly urged to consult the
drug companies' printed instructions before administering any of the drugs
recommended in this book.

British Library Cataloguing in Publication Data
A catalogue record for this book is available from the British Library

Library of Congress Cataloging-in-Publication Data
A catalog record for this book is available from the Library of Congress

ISBN 0 340 76255 1 (pb)

1 2 3 4 5 6 7 8 9 10

Commissioning Editor: Joanna Koster
Production Editor: James Rabson
Production Controller: Iain McWilliams
Cover Designer: Terry Griffiths

Design and Typesetting by J&L Composition Ltd, Filey, North Yorkshire
Printed and bound in Malta by Gutenberg Press Ltd

# Contents

Preface     vii

**Part One:**    Writing Short Essays
General introduction     3
Searching for the best evidence to prepare a topic     7
Structuring your answers     9

**Part Two:**    Practice papers

| | | |
|---|---|---:|
| Paper 1 | Obstetrics | 13 |
| | Gynaecology | 27 |
| Paper 2 | Obstetrics | 41 |
| | Gynaecology | 53 |
| Paper 3 | Obstetrics | 63 |
| | Gynaecology | 75 |
| Paper 4 | Obstetrics | 85 |
| | Gynaecology | 97 |
| Paper 5 | Obstetrics | 109 |
| | Gynaecology | 121 |
| Paper 6 | Obstetrics | 133 |
| | Gynaecology | 143 |
| Paper 7 | Obstetrics | 153 |
| | Gynaecology | 163 |
| Paper 8 | Obstetrics | 173 |
| | Gynaecology | 183 |
| Paper 9 | Obstetrics | 193 |
| | Gynaecology | 203 |
| Paper 10 | Obstetrics | 215 |
| | Gynaecology | 227 |

**Part Three:**   Mock examinations

| | | |
|---|---|---:|
| Paper 11 | Obstetrics | 239 |
| | Gynaecology | 239 |
| Paper 12 | Obstetrics | 240 |
| | Gynaecology | 240 |
| Paper 13 | Obstetrics | 241 |
| | Gynaecology | 241 |
| Paper 14 | Obstetrics | 242 |
| | Gynaecology | 242 |
| Paper 15 | Obstetrics | 243 |
| | Gynaecology | 243 |

# Preface

Practice makes perfect. Everybody reads extensively when preparing for examinations, but with the ongoing changes to examination format and the associated drop in pass rate, it is very likely that candidates will concentrate more on the new components of the MRCOG. They will thus need as much practice as they can get to prepare for the short essay question component of the Part 2 examination.

Our book provides mock question papers along with the outline of the answers that are expected by College examiners and the associated marking scheme. The outline of the answers is easy to put together to form an essay. In this manner, the candidates can assess their status of preparation before the actual examination. Our book is also likely to help with the preparation for the MRCOG OSCE.

The book contains 100 short essay questions with their answers and/or a marking scheme. These will help the candidates to assess themselves during their preparation for the examination. By working their way through the questions, scoring their own marks and obtaining feedback to recognize their strengths and weaknesses, candidates will be able to prepare for the short essay question papers in the Part 2 MRCOG examination with confidence. The book concludes with a set of five mock examinations, giving the candidate an important opportunity to work through further questions without finding the answers readily to hand.

The layout of the questions and answers is designed to be similar in format and degree of difficulty to the questions contained in the outline of answers and the marking scheme used by the Royal College of Obstetricians and Gynaecologists (RCOG). The answers provided are based as much as possible on the current evidence (Cochrane database, systematic reviews and randomized controlled trials) and the RCOG guidelines. In occasional cases, the reader is referred to key review articles that will provide additional and accurate information on a particular topic.

We hope that this book will help you to prepare for the exam and to pass at your first attempt!

*P. Latthe*
*K.S. Khan*
*J.K. Gupta*
*H. Gee*

# Part One
# Writing Short Essays

# Writing Short Essays

## GENERAL INTRODUCTION

Through recent changes, the MRCOG examination is said to have become fairer. It has also become very competitive. Writing a well-constructed, precise essay within the confined time limit has become absolutely essential to pass the written component of the Part 2 MRCOG examination. This means that the candidate, from their vast sea of knowledge, has to bring out those points that will fetch the marks required for passing. This is going to require a lot of practice.

## Introduction to the Exam

There are 10 essay questions divided between two papers. Each paper is allocated 2 h. Thus, each question should be answered in 24 min. Since the marks are divided equally, there is no point in spending more time on one question to the detriment of another.

A structured marking scheme is provided to the examiners marking the papers. This system is fair and reproducible, but is somewhat rigid. To accrue marks, each item on the marking scheme has to be mentioned by the candidate. Thus, thoroughness is of the essence.

The examiners are looking for clarity, a logical sequence to procedures, and a critical appraisal of the options. This means that knowing facts is not enough. The facts have to be organized and weighed to give a reasoned answer to the question. Though it is often overlooked, your own practical experience can be invaluable in this respect.

In spite of the structured marking scheme, the examiners still expect a properly written essay. Planning is essential for two main reasons. It will:

- Help to ensure your answer is complete
- Economize on writing

Time is not usually a limiting factor but the answer has to be no longer than two sides of A4 (49 lines, 300 words). A few minutes spent on grouping facts and determining the sequence in the answer will save time, avoid omitting important facts, help to improve the legibility of handwriting and shorten the answer.

## Why Candidates Fail

Most candidates have enough factual knowledge to pass the examination. They fail because they:

- Do not establish what the question asks
- Do not start at the beginning with the simple stuff

- Get sidetracked
- Miss out important points

The following will help you to avoid these pitfalls and ensure that your knowledge is used to the full.

## Basic Steps to Formulate an Essay Answer

- Read the question
- Brainstorm to ascertain the information
- Group the information
- Plan the answer
- Write
- Review

### Reading the Question

Read the question at least four times:

- First reading
- Identify key words
- Read again – why this question?
- Final reading – verify the gist of the question

The **first reading** gives you the gist of the question. It is possible to latch onto certain words and phrases and then jump to the wrong conclusion. Read carefully without any preconceptions.

It is unlikely that information that is totally irrelevant will be given. Look at the **key words** or terms of the question. Underline them if necessary. They will fall into three categories:

- Instructions
- General information
- Critical data

**Instructions**, not surprisingly, tell you what to do, e.g. evaluate, critically appraise, discuss, etc. **General information** sets the scene. **Critical data** relate to points that are often indicators to the discussion, e.g. parity may be given to lead to discussion over a clinical condition (e.g. fibroids and endometrial cancer tend to occur in women of low parity). Therefore, if the question asks about the investigation of a woman with a uterine mass and parity is given, the answer should include the importance of parity in determining your differential diagnosis. Gestational age carries many connotations: 6–8 weeks, time of presentation for ectopic pregnancy; 24 weeks, legal time of viability; 32 weeks, time when there is a levelling off of death from prematurity; 38 weeks, maturity; 41 weeks, entering gestation when induction and delivery carry benefit. There are other commonly used pieces of critical data, e.g. age, menarche, menopause (pre or post). When they occur, you should ask 'What happens at this time?' or 'What relevance have these circumstances to the main topic?'

**Read the question again** in its entirety. Ask yourself why the question is being posed. Why is it important? Examiners will not set questions for their own sake. They usually tackle everyday or important issues. You may see something you didn't before.

The **final reading** is to ensure you are clear in your own mind what the task is before you. Remember:

- Each point in the question is significant
- Each point has to be addressed
- Do not read unnecessary complexity into the question
- It means what it says

## Brainstorming

You can ask for extra paper for rough working – do so.

Take each key word and piece of critical data and think of its connotations to you in general – whether it appears relevant to the question or not. You can discard bits as needs be. Use 'surgical sieves', e.g. if the question talks about a 'mass' this could be physiological or pathological. If pathological, it could be congenital, inflammatory or neoplastic. If neoplastic, it could be benign or malignant, and if malignant, it could be primary or secondary. This process sparks off connections and other trains of thought, which may be relevant but would have been missed if a narrower approach had been adopted. Another example of a 'surgical sieve' is when you justify a gynaecological patient to be taken to theatre as an emergency – it is justified in case of one of the three Bs: blockade, bleeding or bursting. There will be occasional exceptions to the rule. Know standard classifications for clinical conditions and use correct terminology accordingly.

In your revising, note ballpark data about common conditions, e.g. survival at key gestations, 5-year survival for malignancies or stages of malignancy. Put these figures next to the items to use in support of your arguments. Examiners will not quibble with figures providing they are in the right area – so don't be afraid of using a piece of data you have acquired. It is not wise, however, to make wild guesses.

Statistics and guidance that you will be expected to know can be found in:

- Reports:
  Confidential Enquiry into Stillbirths and Deaths in Infancy (CESDI)
  Confidential Enquiry into Maternal Deaths (CEMD)
  Confidential Enquiry into Perioperative Deaths (CEPOD)
- Guidelines:
  Royal College of Obstetricians and Gynaecologists (RCOG)
  Department of Health (DoH)

## Grouping the Information

You will be able to identify important information and discard the irrelevant. Do so by highlighting and crossing out. Link connected items.

**Planning the Answer**

This is the good bit. Traditionally, there are three parts:

- The introduction or opening gambit
- The body of the answer
- Conclusion

The introduction and conclusion should be very terse. There is not much space and they are not allotted marks. In the **introduction** be brief. Having understood the question and pulled together your knowledge, you should have a clear view of your answer; if not, think a bit more and ask 'Do I understand the question?' and 'Have I the data to answer the question?'

You have grouped your information. Now rearrange it in a flow diagram on your scrap paper so that it flows and give a balanced answer to the question, paying attention to the instructions. This will form the body of the answers. If the question asks for a critical appraisal, then it wants the options available and the pros and cons for each with a decision on the basis of this evidence. This is the bit that gets the marks. Using a structured approach similar to that given at the end of this chapter, you will be able to answer any question that you have never even seen before!

Start at the beginning, even if this seems too simple for a postgraduate examination. Diagnosis requires history, examination and investigations. If you are not certain about including a particular step – e.g. should I establish the gestational age when it is given in the question? – do so, but don't dwell on it. It can often be done in a single sentence, e.g. 'I would check the gestational age by asking about her menstrual history and looking for confirmation from an early ultrasound scan.'

The **conclusion** is the least important of the three. It should just round off. It may be here, for example, that you reach your final decision over the line of management.

**Writing**

Use your plan and stick to it. Write in short, simple sentences. Take your time, and make your writing as legible as possible. Underlining important points can be done, but don't underline everything!

**Reviewing**

Leave a few minutes to read through your answer for silly mistakes. Check that all the important pieces of information in your plan have been included and that you haven't missed any points.

**Key points about formalizing Essay Answers**

- Understand the task
- Gather your knowledge
- Order your knowledge

- Construct your answer logically and clearly
- Write legibly in good English
- Check your answer for accuracy and completeness
- Practise

## SEARCHING FOR THE BEST EVIDENCE TO PREPARE A TOPIC

### Introduction

As in all medical specialities, using the principles of evidence-based medicine is an important part of effective practice. Evidence-based medicine is defined as 'the conscientious, explicit and judicious use of current best evidence in making decisions about the care of individual patients'. It involves several steps, notably formulating a clinical question, searching the literature for relevant clinical articles, evaluating the evidence, and implementing useful findings in clinical practice. This section of the book gives guidance on finding the best available evidence. With ongoing research and constantly updated evidence, it is possible that the reading suggested in this book may not be always the most current. With this in mind, it is important that candidates are able to identify efficiently recent studies that are relevant to the topic being studied. We discuss here three widely used techniques for finding useful evidence: the Cochrane Database of Systematic Reviews, MEDLINE, and the World Wide Web.

### The Cochrane Database of Systematic Reviews

The Cochrane Database of Systematic Reviews (CDSR) contains systematic reviews as part of the Cochrane Library. It is produced by the Cochrane Collaboration, an international network of individuals and institutions that prepare, maintain and disseminate systematic reviews of the effects of health care.

CDSR is an evidence-based medicine resource that includes the full text of the regularly updated systematic reviews of the effects of healthcare. The reviews are presented as two types: regularly updated *Complete Reviews* and those reviews currently under preparation, known as *Protocols*. Systematic reviews are prepared using materials and methods that help to reduce the effects of bias. Reviews are mainly of randomized controlled trials, and results are often combined statistically, with meta-analysis, to increase the power of the findings.

CDSR is unlike other resources in that once a review is published, it will appear in every subsequent issue. Reviews are revised as new research results become available or as errors are identified. As the reviews are updated when new evidence emerges, and mistakes corrected in response to comments and criticisms, the reviews provide probably the best single place to find the latest high-quality evidence.

The other databases included in the Cochrane Library are the York Database of Abstracts of Reviews of Effectiveness (DARE), the Cochrane Review Methodology

Database (CRMD), and the Cochrane Controlled Trials Register (CCTR). The latter is a bibliography of over 100 000 controlled trials, many of which are not listed on MEDLINE or other bibliographical databases.

The Cochrane Library is published quarterly on CD-ROM and the Internet, and is distributed on a subscription basis. Some Internet sites provide access to the Cochrane database, e.g. doctors.net.uk (**http://www.doctors.net.uk**).

## MEDLINE

For almost all searches, most people today use Index Medicus, the catalogue of the United States National Library of Medicine (NLM), and a periodical index to the medical literature. It is available in a printed format, but is better known in its electronic version, MEDLINE.

Index Medicus is a bibliographic listing of references to articles from biomedical journals worldwide. The NLM includes journals that have been assessed as useful by a group including physicians, editors and librarians. Trained literature analysts index the articles. There is an annual Cumulated Index Medicus.

The MEDLINE database is available from different vendors using CD-ROM technology, including Ovid Technologies and Silver Platter Information WinSPIRS. The MEDLINE database is the same, but the commands differ according to the software. MEDLINE can also be accessed via the World Wide Web. For example, the BMA library runs a MEDLINE service for its members, which is available 24 h a day via the Web and also through the Joint Academic Network (JANET).

MEDLINE is also accessible on the Web through PubMed (**http://www.ncbi.nlm.nih.gov/PubMed/**). This is the National Library of Medicine's search service that provides access to over 11 million citations in MEDLINE, Pre-MEDLINE, and other related databases. It also has links to some online journals.

While undoubtedly very useful, MEDLINE has its limitations. Not all medical articles are indexed on MEDLINE, and many that are have been misclassified; article entry depends on human judgement. Many journals (and some sections of indexed journals) are not available. It has been estimated that about 40% of material that should be listed on MEDLINE can be found only by looking through all the journals manually.

## The Internet

Medical research can also be found by searching the World Wide Web directly. This is most easily done by using one or more of the Internet search engines, such as Yahoo (**http://uk.yahoo.com/**), AltaVista (**http://uk.altavista.com/**) or Lycos (**http://www.lycos.co.uk**). For a review of the strengths and weaknesses of each search engine, see the section on search engines at the web site of the Kansas City Public Library (http://www.kcpl.lib.mo.us/search/srchengines.htm). As an alternative to these, there are a number of medical search engines. Some websites such as MEDLINE Pro (**http://MEDLINEpro.com**), allow users to search a number of medical search engines in one go.

It should be remembered that the quality of information on the Web is extremely variable, limiting its use as a serious information source. At the best of times, search engines will find only a fraction of the total literature available on the Web about a particular topic, which is unsurprising since the number of websites continues to grow rapidly. With all search engines, the usefulness of the results will depend largely on the search strategy used, in particular the search entry term(s) used. For example, if the term 'menorrhagia' is used as the search term, the results will be different from those found using the phrase 'heavy periods'. Be aware also that most medical information posted on the Web originates from the USA, and therefore may not always be relevant to candidates preparing for  UK-based examinations such as the MRCOG.

## STRUCTURING YOUR ANSWERS

While preparing the skeleton/outline of your answer, the following provide useful templates for structuring your answers according to the types of questions being asked.

### Critical evaluation

Describe available options.
Discuss pros and cons.
Justify your choice on the basis of evidence.

### Diagnosis
History.
Examination.
Investigations (it is important to indicate which tests have limited value).

### Management
Investigations.
Supportive – includes counselling, information leaflets, support groups.
Medical treatment.
Surgical treatment.

### Risk assessment/Pros and cons
Describe risks and/or benefits.
Justify the management in the light of the risks.
If there are alternatives, give reasons for your choice.
Involving the patient in decision making is important.

### Clinical approach
Diagnosis + management.

### Counselling
Risk assessment + management.

### Screening
Are criteria for screen positive result satisfied?
Screening is not diagnostic!
What are the risks of the diagnosis?
If the diagnosis is confirmed what are the further options in management and are they acceptable to the patient?

### Plan of care for a pregnant patient
Antenatal screening, maternal and fetal monitoring.
Intrapartum management – includes mode of delivery.
Postpartum care, including advice on contraception and preconceptual counselling for the next pregnancy, if indicated.

### Useful reading

Bonnar J. *Recent Advances in Obstetrics and Gynaecology* 20, 21, London: Churchill Livingstone; 1999, 2000.

The Cochrane Library, Issue 3, 2000. Oxford: **http://www.update-software.com**

Farquharson RG. *Vignettes for the MRCOG*, Dinton, Wiltshire: Quay Books; 1998.

James DK, Steer PJ, Weiner CP, Gonik B (eds). *High Risk Pregnancy*, 2nd edn. London: WB Saunders; 1999.

Keirse MJNC, Kanhai HH. Chalmers I. *Effective Care in Pregnancy and Childbirth*, Oxford: Oxford University Press, 1998.

Lewis G, Drife J. *Why Mothers Die – Report on Confidential Enquiries into Maternal Deaths in the UK 1994–1996.* London: HMSO; 1998.

Nelson-Piercy C. *Handbook of Obstetric Medicine*, 1st edn. Oxford: Isis Medical Media; 1997.

RCOG green top guidelines and PACE review articles. RCOG Press: **http://www.rcog.org.uk.**

Shaw RW, Soutter WP, Stanton SI. *Gynaecology*, 2nd edn. London: Churchill Livingstone; 1997.

Stirratt GM. *Aids to Obstetrics in Gynaecology for MRCOG*, 4th edn. London: Churchill Livingstone; 1998.

Studd J. *Progress in Obstetrics and Gynaecology 14*, London: Churchill Livingstone; 2000.

# Part Two

# **Practice Papers**

# PAPER 1 OBSTETRICS

1. A 30-year-old primigravida attends for an ultrasound scan because she has been found to have large for dates uterus at her 28-week visit. The fetus is diagnosed to have scalp oedema, ascites and bilateral pleural effusion. Discuss critically the causes and investigations of this case, who has no abnormal red cell antibodies.

2. Discuss critically the alternatives for the management of fetal death at 29 weeks gestation.

3. What is bacterial vaginosis? Discuss its diagnosis and significance in gynaecological and obstetric practice.

4. Debate the evidence for the various tocolytic agents curently in use.

5. Justify the statement, 'Intrapartum electronic fetal monitoring should be restricted to high-risk pregnancies'.

1. A 30-year-old primigravida attends for an ultrasound scan because she has been found to have large for dates uterus at her 28-week visit. The fetus is diagnosed to have scalp oedema, ascites and bilateral pleural effusion. Discuss critically the causes and investigations of this case, who has no abnormal red cell antibodies.

The diagnosis in this case is non-immune hydrops fetalis (NIFH). It is the result of a heterogeneous group of conditions. Cardiovascular malformations, arrhythmia and neoplasm cause about 20% of NIFH.

The other important causes are chromosomal anomalies (trisomy 21, 18, 13 and Turner's syndrome), haematological disorders such as alpha thalassaemia, pulmonary malformations, genitourinary anomalies, intrauterine infections, cystic hygroma. Approximately one-third of the cases are of idiopathic origin.

Complete maternal health history, including determination of ethnicity, previous history of jaundice, and exposure to infection, should be taken.

Investigations of infectious exposure (parvovirus, syphilis, rubella, cytomegalovirus, toxoplasma, echovirus and coxsackievirus) should be carried out. Maternal blood tests should include glucose screen, haemoglobin electrophoresis, syphilis serology, Kleihauer test, and glucose 6-phosphatase dehydrogenase activity. If congenital heart block is diagnosed, then it is useful to test for anti-Ro and anti-La antibodies.

Detailed ultrasound to look for structural anomalies such as skeletal dysplasia, and genitourinary, gastrointestinal and cord abnormalities is carried out by an expert in fetal medicine. Fetal echocardiography and cardiac Doppler studies to rule out cardiac abnormalities must be done.

Cordocentesis is carried out for blood count, fetal karyotype, viral titres, blood gases, cultures, liver function (including serum albumin) and metabolic testing, (urea and electrolytes), and haemoglobin electrophoresis. Amniocentesis for viral culture and karyotyping is another alternative.

In case of stillbirth or neonatal death, postmortem can provide vital clues to aetiology.

## Answer key and marking scheme

The diagnosis is non-immune fetal hydrops.                                          1 mark

The different causative factors include cardiac, haematological, pulmonary,          1 mark
gastrointestinal malformations, neoplastic causes and infections.

The other important causes are chromosomal anomalies (trisomy 21, 18, 13             1 mark
and Turner's syndrome).
About 20–30% of cases are idiopathic in origin.

Maternal history including exposure to possible teratogens.                          1 mark
Maternal blood tests: full blood count and film, viral screen (booking serum
can be tested for antibodies against syphilis, cytomegalovirus, toxoplasmosis,
Herpes simplex, respiratory syncytial virus and HPVB19).

Haemoglobin electrophoresis, Kleihauer–Betke test, glucose screen.                   1 mark
Anti-Ro and anti-La antibodies if congenital heart block is diagnosed.

Detailed fetal ultrasound.                                                           1 mark
Fetal echocardiography and cardiac Doppler studies.

Refer to fetal medicine centre for expert interdisciplinary management and           1 mark
further investigations.

Cordocentesis for karyotyping, viral screen (TORCH and HPVB19), urea                 1 mark
and electrolytes, full blood count, blood film and liver function tests.

Amniocentesis for viral culture and karyotyping is another alternative.              1 mark

Postmortem examination in cases of stillbirth or neonatal death may provide          1 mark
vital clues to possible aetiology.

## Suggested reading

Forouzan I. Hydrops fetalis: recent advances. *Obstet Gynecol Surv* 1997; 52(2): 130–8.

2. Discuss critically the alternatives for the management of fetal death at 29 weeks gestation.

---

The woman should be given the options with detailed information (preferably by a consultant) and the time to decide what she wants. Her options are to choose between expectant and active care.

There are no overt benefits or hazards for the induction of labour over expectant care. The advantages and disadvantages are related mostly to their psychological and emotional effects.

For some women carrying the dead fetus permits them a feeling of closeness that is lost after birth. If induction of labour is decided hastily without adequate consultation with parents, it may be seen as a sign of compensating for guilt.

The main advantage of expectant care is non-intervention. The woman does not need to come into the hospital and undergo procedures that might be more risky than non-intervention.

The disadvantages of expectant care are psychological stress and the unpredictably long time that the woman may need to go into spontaneous labour. Occasionally, the woman and her relatives have the misconception that the dead fetus is poisoning the mother's blood.

The only physical risk of conservative management is potential of increased risk of coagulopathy, which is most likely to occur in cases of abruptio placentae. It is rarely associated with other causes of fetal death. The hypofibrinogenaemia is rarely significant during the first 4–5 weeks after fetal death.

The advantage of active policy is that it may be preferable for many women to end a pregnancy that has lost its purpose. Postmortem studies are easier in fresh stillbirth than a macerated stillbirth. It is also more convenient because of its predictability.

The disadvantage relates to the means used for the induction. If active policy is chosen, the prostaglandin can be administered by the vaginal, intra-amniotic or extra-amniotic routes. In spite of their efficacy, all the methods have drawbacks, such as fever, rigors, increased pain and need for analgesia

Tender loving care, pain relief, named midwives on the labour ward, time with the baby after delivery, photographs, prints, consent for postmortem examination, organization of burial/cremation according to the parents' wishes, and lactation suppression and contraception are part of the management in both policies.

The general practitioner and the community midwife need to be informed. The investigations to search for the cause for intrauterine death, such as karyotyping, diabetic screen, and thrombophilia screening, are carried out, and a visit after 6 weeks to see the consultant is organized before the woman is discharged.

## Answer key and marking scheme

*A good candidate will discuss the advantages and disadvantages associated with the two options, expectant and active care. Do not forget to enlist steps in management common to both alternatives.*

There are no overt benefits or hazards for the induction of labour over expectant care.                                                                    1 mark
The advantages and disadvantages relate to their psychological and emotional effects on the woman and her partner.

### Expectant management
The main disadvantage of expectant care is non-intervention                 1 mark

The disadvantages of expectant care are psychological stress, the            1 mark
unpredictability of the events, and increased risk of coagulopathy.

### Active management
The advantage of active policy is that it may be a preferable option to the  1 mark
pregnant woman to end the pregnancy that has lost its purpose.

Postmortem diagnosis is easier to reach in fresh stillbirth.                 1 mark

It is more predictable than awaiting spontaneous onset of events.            1 mark

If induction of labour is decided with little input from parents, it may be seen  1 mark
as a search for quick solution.

Prostaglandins can be administered by various routes, but despite their      1 mark
efficacy they all have drawbacks, such as fever, rigors, increased pain and need
 for analgesia.

The intra- and postpartum care is similar in both alternatives: tender loving  1 mark
care, adequate analgesia, photographs, prints, consent for postmortem
examination, investigate for possible causes and inform patient's family doctor
and midwife.

The investigations to search for the cause for intrauterine death, such as   1 mark
karyotyping, diabetic screen, and thrombophilia screening are carried out.
Visit after 6 weeks to see consultant is organized before the woman is
discharged.

## Suggested reading
Keirse MJNC, Kanhai HH, Chalmers I. Fetal death, in *Effective Care in Pregnancy and Childbirth*. Oxford: Oxford University Press; 1998. pp. 183–90.

3. What is bacterial vaginosis? Discuss its diagnosis and significance in gynaecological and obstetric practice.

Bacterial vaginosis (BV) is a polymicrobial condition in the vagina where there is a fall in the number of lactobacilli and rise in the vaginal pH. The number of anaerobic bacteria such as *Gardnerella vaginalis*, mobiluncus species, mycoplasma, ureaplasma and bacteroides increases. BV contributes to 10–30% of all the cases of symptomatic vaginal discharge.

The diagnosis comprises tests such as homogenous vaginal discharge with pH more than 5, positive amine whiff test, and clue cells on wet microscopy (Hillier and Holmes' composite criteria).

BV is linked to sexual activity. The partner does not require screening. BV is treated easily with metronidazole or clindamycin.

There is an association of BV with the development of vault infections and haematomas following hysterectomy or other vaginal surgery. Vault haematoma causes pain, pyrexia, restricted mobility, predisposition to venous thrombosis and sometimes pelvic abscess. It has also been associated with cervical intraepithelial neoplasia, urinary tract infection, lower abdominal pain, menorrhagia and pelvic inflammatory disease in a few studies. It has also been associated with increased risk of HIV acquisition.

BV has been implicated in recurrent miscarriage. Presence of BV in the first trimester of pregnancy is a risk factor for second trimester miscarriage. It does not affect conception, but it has been associated with an increased risk of miscarriage in the first trimester in women undergoing *in vitro* fertilization, independent of other risk factors.

BV is associated with preterm premature rupture of membranes. It is associated with a five-fold increase in preterm birth when detected before 16 weeks gestation. Post-caesarean wound infections are increased. It has been connected with postpartum endometritis and secondary postpartum haemorrhage.

Mothers likely to benefit from 'screen and treat' approaches include those with the highest concentrations of genital anaerobes and mycoplasmas, women with prior preterm birth or who have low body mass index (BMI <20 kg/m$^2$), and those with evidence of endometritis before pregnancy.

## Answer key and marking scheme

*A good candidate should define the condition, the criteria for diagnosis, its association with disorders in obstetrics and gynaecology with a proposition for selective screening.*

### Definition
Bacterial vaginosis (BV) is a clinical condition caused by replacement of the normal lactobacillus species in the vagina with high concentrations of characteristic sets of aerobic and anaerobic bacteria (*Gardnerella*, ureaplasma, bacteroides and mobiluncus species).      1 mark

**Diagnosis** requires the presence of three out of four of the following:      2 marks

- Vaginal fluid pH >4.5
- Homogenous white adherent vaginal discharge
- Clue cells on wet mount
- Fishy odour on addition of 10% KOH

(*½ mark for each point mentioned*)

### Gynaecology
Association with post-hysterectomy vaginal cuff infection, vault haematoma.      1 mark

BV has been associated with pelvic inflammatory disease, urinary tract infection and, rarely, pelvic abscess, menorrhagia and lower abdominal pain.      1 mark

According to some studies, women with BV have more than twice the incidence of cervical dysplasia and abnormal cervical biopsies than compared to women without BV.      1 mark

### Obstetrics
BV has been implicated in recurrent second trimester miscarriage and preterm labour.      1 mark

Preterm premature rupture of membranes is associated with presence of BV.      1 mark

Risk of postpartum endometritis and secondary postpartum haemorrhage as well as post-caesarean wound infections is increased because of infection with bacterial vaginosis during pregnancy.      1 mark

### Selective screening
Those women who are at higher risk of preterm birth, with a history of recurrent miscarriage, or are symptomatic must be screened and treated with metronidazole or clindamycin.      1 mark

## Suggested reading

Brocklehurst P, Hannah M, McDonald H. Interventions for treating bacterial vaginosis in pregnancy [systematic review], Cochrane Pregnancy and Childbirth Group, in The Cochrane Library, Issue 3, 2000. Oxford: Update software.

Soper DE. Gynaecologic sequelae of bacterial vaginosis. *Int J Gynaecol Obstet* 1999; 67(1): S25–8.

Woodrow N, Lamont RF. Bacterial vaginosis: its importance in obstetrics. *Br J Hosp Med* 1998; 59(6): 447–9.

4. Debate the evidence for the various tocolytic agents currently in use.

Tocolytic use in preterm labour has not been shown to improve perinatal outcomes, but the various agents used do delay delivery by 24–48 h, which can be used to administer steroids and effect *in utero* transfer if necessary.

Beta agonists confer significant benefit in terms of reducing number of deliveries within 24–48 h, although no benefit has been noted in reducing respiratory distress syndrome (RDS) or severe respiratory problems or perinatal deaths.

Women whose labour is initially arrested with tocolytics are at high risk for recurrent preterm labour, rehospitalization, and need for recurrent intravenous tocolytics. Maintenance tocolytic therapy has been used to reduce the risk of recurrent preterm labour in such women. Oral tablets, cutaneous patches and subcutaneous pumps are some of the routes used. However, the effectiveness of these therapies in decreasing the risk of preterm birth or low birth weight or increasing the interval until birth cannot be established.

Efficacy of nifedipine in suppressing preterm labour is possibly better than beta agonists with similar results as beta agonists in prolonging labour. There is no improvement in perinatal mortality (in common with beta agonists). Better side-effects profile and no deleterious effects on the fetus might make it more preferable to the beta agonists.

Antiprostaglandins, such as indomethacin, reduce preterm delivery within 48 h and 7 days, and show a trend towards reducing respiratory morbidity and perinatal deaths. Significant maternal and fetal side effects have been documented, and making it less favourable for clinical use.

Magnesium sulphate has shown to be ineffective in reducing any adverse outcomes. It is also associated with some serious side effects, such as pulmonary oedema, respiratory depression, cardiac arrest and death.

Oxytocin antagonist (e.g. atosiban) are available. Recent, large, multicentre trials show these to be comparably effective to ritodrine with regards to delaying labour, but with better side-effects profile. Atosiban is effective over 28 weeks, but efficacy under 28 weeks is inconclusive.

Cyclo-oxygenase 2 (COX-2) inhibitors and nitric oxide donors have not been assessed adequately in large clinical trials.

## Answer key and marking scheme

*A good candidate will discuss the evidence regarding benefits and side effects of beta agonists, calcium channel blockers, magnesium sulphate, antiprostaglandins, oxytocin antagonists and nitric oxide.*

Tocolytics confer significant benefit in terms of reducing number of deliveries within 24–48 h.

1 mark

This time can be used effectively for administration of steroids and *in utero* transfer, if necessary, to special care baby unit.

1 mark

No benefit is noted in reducing severe respiratory problems or perinatal deaths.

1 mark

### Beta agonists
Use of beta agonists is associated with high levels of maternal side effects especially pulmonary oedema.

The effectiveness of the maintenance tocolytic therapies in decreasing the risk of preterm birth or low birth weight or increasing the interval until birth is unproven.

1 mark

### Calcium channel blockers
Efficacy of nifedipine in suppressing preterm labour is as good as, or even possibly better than, beta agonists.

1 mark

No improvement in perinatal mortality (in common with beta agonists).
Better side-effects profile.
No deleterious effects on fetus.

1 mark

### Indomethacin
Indomethacin reduces preterm delivery within 48 h and 7 days, and shows a trend towards reducing RDS and perinatal deaths.
Significant maternal and fetal side-effects have been documented like premature closure of ductus arteriosus and adverse fetal renal function.

1 mark

**Magnesium sulphate**: there is not enough evidence to show that magnesium maintenance therapy is effective in preventing preterm birth after an episode of threatened preterm labour.

1 mark

**Oxytocin antagonist** (atosiban): recent, large, multicentre trials show this drug to be comparably effective to ritodrine with regards to delaying labour, but with a vastly better side-effects profile.

1 mark

Atosiban is effective over 28 weeks, but efficacy under 28 weeks was inconclusive.

COX-2 inhibitors and nitric oxide donors have better side-effect profile than          1 mark
Indomethacin but are awaiting large clinical trials for definitive evidence.

## Suggested reading

Crowther CA, Moore V. Magnesium for preventing preterm birth after threatened preterm labour [Cochrane Review], in The Cochrane Library, Issue 3, 2000. Oxford: Update software

RCOG. *Green Top Guidelines No. 1A*. London: Royal College of Obstetricians and Gynaecologists; 1995.

RCOG. *Green Top Guidelines No. 7*. London: Royal College of Obstetricians and Gynaecologists; 1996.

Smith P, Anthony J, Johanson R. Nifedipine in pregnancy. *Br J Obstet Gynaecol* 2000; 107: 299–307.

5.  Justify the statement, 'Intrapartum electronic fetal monitoring should be restricted to high-risk pregnancies.'

Intrapartum electronic fetal monitoring (EFM) is aimed at minimizing fetal demise and long-term consequences, such as cerebral palsy.

Evidence to date is that in low risk labour caesarean section rate is higher in the electronically monitored group as are vaginal operative deliveries. The higher operative interventions then reflect in higher rates of infectious morbidity postpartum. There is no difference in perinatal mortality, 1-min Apgar scores <4 or 5-min <7, or neonatal admission rate.

There was a 50% reduction in neonatal seizures in the electronically monitored group, but follow-up data suggest that the seizures prevented are not those associated with long-term neurological impairments. Intrapartum death is prevented equally effectively by the two modalities when prompt action is taken on prompt recognition of fetal heart rate abnormalities by either method.

Whilst some women find electronic monitoring reassuring, others report discomfort and limited mobility, and are worried about the possible damage to the baby's scalp with the internal electrode. Women in the electronically monitored group tend to be left alone for longer periods.

Continuous electronic fetal monitoring provides more accurate information of the fetal heart rate, but its interpretation can be subjective and it requires regular training and updates of personnel. It has potential for technical or mechanical failure.

In women who have antenatal and intrapartum risk factors (like postmaturity, fetal growth restriction, pre-eclampsia, oxytocin induction or augmentation), EFM is recommended on the basis of well controlled trials.

Hence the current consensus is that continuous electronic monitoring should be restricted to high-risk pregnancies. The form of fetal monitoring should be discussed with the mother in low-risk labours to ascertain her wishes. Women should be allowed to make informed choices regarding this aspect of care by access to evidence based information.

## Answer key and marking scheme

*A good candidate will discuss the objective of monitoring, the pros and cons of continuous monitoring, and the rationale behind the proposition of restricting continuous monitoring to high-risk pregnancies.*

### Objective of fetal monitoring
Antenatal and intrapartum fetal monitoring are aimed at avoiding fetal          1 mark
 demise and long-term consequences, such as cerebral palsy.

### Pros
EFM is shown to be useful in reducing adverse fetal and neonatal sequel in
high-risk pregnancies                                                          1 mark

There is a 50% reduction in neonatal seizures in the electronically monitored   1 mark
group, but follow-up data suggest that the seizures prevented are not those
associated with long-term neurological impairments.

Many women find electronic monitoring reassuring.                              1 mark

### Cons
Caesarean section and vaginal operative delivery rates are higher in the        1 mark
 electronically monitored group. This translates into higher infection rate in
the mother.

There is no difference in perinatal mortality in low-risk labour.              1 mark

There is no difference in 1-min Apgar scores <4 or  5-min Apgar scores
<7 or neonatal admission rate.

Women in the electronically monitored group tend to be left alone for longer    1 mark
periods.

Some women report discomfort and limited mobility, and are worried about        1 mark
the possible damage to the baby's scalp with the internal electrode.

It is at risk of technical or mechanical faults. It is costly for maintenance.  1 mark
The interpretation can be subjective and requires training of the personnel
using it.

### Rationale                                                                  1 mark
Given the fact that there is no benefit to fetus or mother in a low-risk
labour, on balance, the proposition to limit electronic monitoring to
high-risk pregnancy is reasonable. Nevertheless the form of fetal monitoring
should be discussed with low-risk mothers and their choice respected.

## Suggested reading

Thacker SB, Stroup DF. Continuous electronic heart rate monitoring for fetal assessment during labour, in The Cochrane Library, Issue 3, 2000. Oxford: Update software.

# PAPER 1: GYNAECOLOGY

1. A 19-year-old university student is referred by her GP at 7 weeks gestation with request for termination of pregnancy. How will you manage her once the decision to terminate the pregnancy has been made?

2. Summarize the non-contraceptive uses of the levonorgestrel intrauterine system.

3. A 34-year-old woman, whose mother and sister suffered from breast and ovarian cancer, respectively, is concerned about her risk of cancer. On further questioning, it is revealed that her grandmother also died of ovarian cancer. She has no children. What are her risks and further management options?

4. A 21-year-old woman is referred by her GP with infrequent menstrual periods and hirsutism. She has a body mass index of 32 and is diagnosed to have polycystic ovaries. She wishes to know the implications of this disorder. Discuss the issues on which you will counsel her.

5. Discuss the role of endometrial ablation in the treatment of menorrhagia. How will you advise the patient regarding this procedure?

1. A 19-year-old university student is referred by her GP at 7 weeks gestation with request for termination of pregnancy. How will you manage her once the decision to terminate the pregnancy has been made?

---

The procedure should, ideally be done within a week of the appointment. At the same time, of course, adequate time should be allowed for the girl to consider her decision. One must make sure that the abortion certificate is completed and signed. Verbal advice must be supported by accurate, impartial, printed information, which the patient can understand and may take away and read before the procedure.

To minimize the risk of post-abortion infection, screening for lower genital tract organisms and treatment of positive cases should be carried out. The other option is universal prophylaxis with metronidazole 1 g rectally at the time of abortion plus doxycycline 100 mg twice daily for 7 days.

Determine ABO and rhesus blood groups, and give anti-D following the procedure if the woman is rhesus negative.

She should be given the option to choose between medical and surgical methods of abortion.

For medical termination of pregnancy (TOP), mifepristone (200 mg orally) followed by prostaglandin (gemeprost 1 mg vaginally or misoprostol 800 µg vaginally) 36–48 h later is given. It is effective in 95% of cases at this gestation. Misoprostol is unlicensed for abortion procedure, but can be administered if the patient is informed properly and her consent obtained.

Suction-evacuation can be done under general or local anaesthesia as a day-case procedure. Cervical priming with prostaglandin reduces the risk of cervical damage.

Before she is discharged following abortion, the patient should have agreed a future contraceptive plan and should be offered contraceptive supplies. The chosen method of contraception should be initiated immediately following abortion.

On discharge the patient should be given a letter that gives sufficient information about the procedure. A follow-up appointment within 2 weeks of the procedure should be offered to her. Facilities for additional counselling if required should be made available to her.

## Answer key and marking scheme:

*A good candidate will discuss the investigations and management systematically in preoperative, intra-operative and postoperative phases.*

### Preoperative
Make arrangement for her to have TOP within 7 days if possible because of the lower incidence of complications at earlier gestational age.                                             1 mark

Information leaflets should be made available to the patient, which she may take away and read before the procedure.                                             1 mark

Screening for infection and its treatment or universal antibiotic prophylaxis.          2 marks

Determine ABO and rhesus group and give anti-D to Rh-negative non-sensitized patient.                                             1 mark

### Operative
Medical TOP with mifepristone followed by Cervagem or misoprostol (unlicensed) is an alternative to surgery.                                             1 mark

Suction-evacuation under general or local anaesthesia can be done as a day-case procedure.                                             1 mark

Cervical priming before surgical TOP is desirable.                                             1 mark

### Postoperative
Discuss and agree on a future contraceptive plan. Contraceptives supplies should be offered if required.                                             1 mark

Offer a follow-up appointment and additional counselling if necessary.          1 mark

## Suggested reading
RCOG. *Guideline No. 11: Induced Abortion*. London: RCOG Press; 1997.

2. Summarize the non-contraceptive uses of the levonorgestrel intrauterine system.

The levonorgestrel intrauterine system (LNG-IUS) has made a major impact on the treatment of menorrhagia. In cases of dysfunctional uterine bleeding (DUB), it has been shown to cause a 97% reduction in the amount of menstrual blood loss (MBL) after 1 year of use. The haemoglobin and serum ferritin concentrations increase significantly and up to 35% of the women become amenorrhoeic. The LNG-IUS is a simple, effective and cheap treatment for DUB, and is an alternative to both hysterectomy and endometrial ablation, with the advantage of preserving fertility.

Several studies have reported relief from dysmenorrhoea after use of Mirena. Although the device is not usually prescribed solely for this purpose, this may be considered in cases where other treatment has failed and pelvic pathology has been excluded.

Women with fibroids may benefit from the LNG-IUS. There is evidence to suggest a reduced incidence of fibroids and fibroid-related surgery in LNG-IUS users.

Adenomyosis causes progressive menorrhagia and dysmenorrhoea in middle-aged women. Use of the LNG-IUS is associated with marked relief from adenomyosis-associated menorrhagia.

The LNG-IUS can be an effective way of providing continuous progestogen during hormone replacement therapy (HRT), especially for perimenopausal women who suffer from DUB and also require contraception. The bleeding problems are least common and the compliance rates highest in women whose progesterone arm of HRT is LNG-IUS.

The LNG-IUS may be useful in women suffering from premenstrual syndrome (PMS). For women with severe PMS, the only effective cure is total hysterectomy with bilateral salpingo-oophorectomy. Many women find a trial with a continuous oestrogen regimen of oestradiol patches or implants and continuous slow low-dose release of progestogen from the LNG-IUS, effective enough to avoid hysterectomy.

Use of Mirena is associated with reduced incidence of pelvic infection and ectopic pregnancy compared with a copper device. In selected cases of endometrial hyperplasia, the LNG-IUS may be used as it releases progestogen at the site of pathology and is known to achieve regressive changes involving the whole endometrial thickness. Further research is awaited in this field, including the risk of relapse after removal of the device.

Tamoxifen used to treat breast cancer is known to increase the risks of hyperplasia, polyps and cancer. When used in conjunction with LNG-IUS, this risk could potentially be reduced. If trials confirm this, the LNG-IUS would be the contraceptive method of choice in premenopausal women using tamoxifen.

## Answer key and marking scheme

Menorrhagia – 97% reduction in the amount of menstrual blood loss at the   1 mark
end of 1 year, rise in haemoglobin and ferritin concentration.
Oligomenorrhoea in the majority and amenorrhoea in 35%.

Reduction in the rate of hysterectomy and endometrial ablation carried out for   1 mark
menorrhagia.

Dysmenorrhoea can be improved in 80% of cases.   1 mark

Reduced incidence and growth of fibroids.   1 mark

Severe premenstrual syndrome – along with oestradiol implants or continuous   1 mark
high-dose oestradiol skin patches. A good alternative for hysterectomy with
bilateral salpingo-oophorectomy.

Reduction in the risk of pelvic inflammatory disease and ectopic pregnancy   1 mark
compared with copper devices (and compared with non-users of
contraception for ectopic pregnancy).

Adenomyosis-symptomatic improvement.   1 mark

Progestogen arm of HRT.   1 mark

Use in selected cases of endometrial hyperplasia in research setting.   1 mark

In conjunction with tamoxifen – studies are currently being conducted to   1 mark
establish the effectiveness of the LNG-IUS in preventing and treating
hyperplasia induced by tamoxifen.

## Suggested reading

Lethaby AE, Cooke I, Rees M. Progesterone/progestogen releasing intrauterine systems versus either placebo or any other medication for heavy menstrual bleeding [Cochrane Review], in The Cochrane Library, Issue 4, 2000. Oxford: Update software.

Sturridge F, Guillebaud J. Gynaecological aspects of the levonorgestrel-releasing intrauterine system. Br J Obstet Gynaecol, 1997; 104: 285–9.

Van den Hurk PJ, O'Brien S. Non-contraceptive use of the levonorgestrel releasing intrauterine system. The Obstetrician and Gynaecologist 1999; 1(1): 13–16.

3.    A 34-year-old woman, whose mother and sister suffered from breast and ovarian cancer, respectively, is concerned about her risk of cancer. On further questioning, it is revealed that her grandmother also died of ovarian cancer. She has no children. What are her risks and further management options?

She is at high risk for development of both breast and ovarian cancer. It is likely that a mutation predisposing to cancer is being transmitted through this family, most probably in an autosomal dominant fashion.

A mutation in BRCA1 is likely. Women having BRCA1 or BRCA2 gene mutation have a lifetime risk of development of breast cancer 10 times higher than the general population (80% v. 8%). The patient's own risks can be quantified when her carrier status is clear.

The patient's family should be offered genetic counselling and mutation testing of BRCA1 and BRCA2. If affected family members are found to have a mutation, then the others can be offered predictive testing. There are some major limitations to genetic testing that include important implications on financial and insurance policies. Complicated moral issues are raised for all family members if a mutated gene is identified in the family.

If the patient's test is negative, she still has a background lifetime risk of 1 in 12 for breast cancer and 1 in 80 for ovarian cancer. Counselling should include the fact that variable penetrance of mutations makes risk assessment difficult. Psychological counselling concerning carrier status is a part of multidisciplinary management in genetic testing.

If she does not undergo mutation testing, or if she tests positive then she should be taught to do breast self-examination every month. She should also be offered screening with 1–2-yearly mammograms. For ovarian cancer screening, yearly transvaginal scans and serum CA-125 estimation can be offered. However, she should be warned that there is no evidence that this screening reduces mortality for ovarian cancer.

Oral contraceptives, despite the concern that they might increase the risk of breast cancer, have been shown to decrease the risk of ovarian cancer in the general population by as much as 60%. She can use them if she is not planning for a family.

Tamoxifen is another strategy under consideration as chemoprophylaxis for breast cancer, but it is associated with several adverse side effects and an acceptable risk : benefit ratio has not yet been established.

A more radical surgical option for those who test positive is bilateral mastectomy with reconstruction. Efficacy of prophylactic mastectomy in reducing the risk of breast cancer varies from 1 to 19%.

Despite the fact that there are insufficient data substantiating its efficacy, bilateral oophorectomy (laparoscopic if possible) is provided as an option during counselling. It is a fact that prophylactic oophorectomy cannot prevent the development of primary peritoneal carcinoma. In-depth counselling and preparation is vital. The patient should be aware that there are uncertainties over ongoing risks of malignancy and hormone replacement in these women.

## Answer key and marking scheme

*A good candidate will discuss the likelihood of BRCA1 and BRCA2 mutation, and offer screening to affected family members. If they are positive, then unaffected relatives can be tested. The screen positive members can be offered yearly surveillance mammography, transvaginal ultrasound, CA-125 levels, use of combined pills, tamoxifen and surgical options of bilateral mastectomy and oophorectomy. (Be on the lookout for the latest developments in this field as this information may become outdated rapidly.)*

### Prognosis
A mutation in BRCA1 is likely. These carry overall breast and ovarian cancer risks of up to 40–45% by the age of 70 years. The risk in BRCA2 carriers for ovarian cancer is 25%.

1 mark

### Genetic screening
The patient's family should be offered genetic counselling and mutation testing of BRCA1 and BRCA2.
If affected family members are found to have a mutation, then the others, including the patient, can be offered predictive testing.

1 mark

Limitations – important implications on financial and insurance policies. Moral questions are raised for all family members if a mutated gene is identified in the family.

1 mark

### Screen negative
If the patient's test is negative, she still has a background lifetime risk of 1 in 12 for breast cancer and 1in 80 for ovarian cancer.

1 mark

### Screen positive
If she is positive, then various strategies for screening/management are proposed.

### Supportive management
If she does not undergo mutation testing, or if she tests positive, then she should be taught to do breast self-examination every month. Mammograms yearly.

1 mark

Yearly CA-125, pelvic examination and/or transvaginal ultrasound ( no evidence that mortality from ovarian cancer is reduced).

1 mark

Psychological counselling concerning carrier status is a part of multidisciplinary management in genetic testing.

1 mark

### Medical treatment
Chemoprophylaxis – combined oral contraceptives, tamoxifen.

1 mark

**Surgical options for screen positive women**
Bilateral mastectomy and reconstruction. 1 mark

Bilateral oophorectomy when family is completed (pros and cons of hormone replacement need to be discussed). 1 mark

## Suggested reading

Fasouliotis SJ, Schenker JG. BRCA1 and BRCA2 gene mutations: decision-making dilemmas concerning testing and management. *Obstet Gynecol Surv* 2000; 55(6): 373–84.

4. A 21-year-old woman is referred by her GP with infrequent menstrual periods and hirsutism. She has a body mass index of 32 and is diagnosed to have polycystic ovaries. She wishes to know the implications of this disorder. Discuss the issues on which you will counsel her.

Around one in five women have polycystic ovaries. The symptoms of polycystic ovaries are a sequel of the loss of ovulation. The symptoms can range from dysfunctional bleeding to amenorrhoea, hirsutism and obesity. Some women might experience acne and scalp hair loss. Subfertility can be a problem due to anovulation. Women who conceive have a higher risk of miscarriage than average because of the raised luteinizing hormone (LH) levels.

Obese, anovulatory women with hyperinsulinaemia are probably at increased risk of coronary heart disease and hypertension because of abnormal lipid profile. The risk of diabetes mellitus in patients with hyperinsulinaemia is higher than in the background population. The risk for hypertension and other cardiovascular risks are also higher. There is an increased risk of endometrial hyperplasia and even malignancy. The risk of breast cancer may be higher, but this is not proven.

Simple weight loss often restores ovulation, so it is encouraged. Stopping smoking, and maintaining a high-fibre, low-fat, low-sugar diet at a young age may help reduce the cardiovascular risks in later life. Some women are at risk of psychological problems. They require sensitive, honest and reassuring discussion, and referral to a clinical psychologist or psychotherapist as deemed appropriate.

Non-pharmacological treatment for hirsutism includes waxing, bleaching, shaving, depilation and electrolysis.

Combined oral pills are recommended until childbearing is desired. Such treatment suppresses ovarian function, reducing androgen levels, controls skin manifestations, protects the endometrium, induces regular withdrawal bleeds, and is a safe contraceptive. If hirsutism is a problem then a pill containing cyproterone acetate (Dianette) is an option. If combined pills are contraindicated or not desirable, cyclical treatment with progestogens is an alternative.

If infertility treatment is required, clomiphene citrate can restore ovulation if weight loss alone is insufficient. *In vitro* fertilization is occasionally offered to those who fail to conceive with other treatment.

There is no role for ovarian drilling for symptoms other than infertility. It might also help to reduce the risk of miscarriage by lowering LH levels.

Information leaflets back up the information given during counselling. The names and addresses of the support groups are provided.

## Answer key and marking scheme

*A good candidate will inform the patient of the clinical implications of polycystic ovaries. The treatment offered is structured into supportive, medical and surgical options. Investigations are not necessary as the diagnosis is made clear in the question. Do not forget the psychological support!*

**Potential clinical consequences of polycystic ovaries**

Menstrual bleeding disorders from amenorrhoea to dysfunctional uterine bleeding.
Hirsutism, acne, oily skin, temporal baldness.
1 mark

Infertility, higher risk of miscarriage.
1 mark

Increased risk of endometrial cancer and perhaps breast cancer.
Increased risk of cardiovascular disease, including hypertension.
1 mark

Increased risk of obesity and diabetes mellitus in patients with hyperinsulinemia.
1 mark

**Supportive treatment**

Encourage weight loss: normalizing weight will reduce most of the risks associated with polycystic ovaries (PCO).
Stopping smoking, and maintaining a high-fibre, low-fat, low-sugar diet at a young age may help reduce the cardiovascular risks in later life.
1 mark

The need for psychological support is addressed depending upon the individual patient. Reassurance is important.
Information leaflets, support groups.
1 mark

**Medical treatment**

Combined oral contraceptive pills suppress the ovaries, reduce androgen levels, control skin manifestations of PCO, protect the endometrium, induce regular withdrawal bleeds and are a safe contraceptive.
A pill containing cyproterone acetate (Dianette) can be used in the presence of hirsutism.
1 mark

For the patient who does not wish pregnancy or to take oral contraceptive pills, but wants a regular bleeding pattern, medroxyprogesterone acetate 10 mg daily for the first 10 days of each month is an alternative.
1 mark

For PCO related infertility, medical induction with clomiphene is done in the first instance. If tablets fail, gonadotrophins are the next drugs of choice.
1 mark

*In vitro* fertilization is occasionally offered to women with PCO when other treatments have failed.

**Surgical treatment**
There is no role for ovarian drilling, unless infertility is the complaint and                    1 mark
medical induction has failed.

## Suggested reading

Taylor AE. Polycystic ovary syndrome. *Endocrinol Metab Clin North Am* 1998; 27(4): 877–902.

5. Discuss the role of endometrial ablation in the treatment of menorrhagia. How will you advise the patient regarding this procedure?

The severity of symptoms such as anaemia and impairment of social and personal life determines requirement for treatment. Endometrial ablation is offered if the other alternatives of treatment, i.e. medical and progesterone intrauterine system, have failed or have been declined by the patient.

The technique is most suitable for dysfunctional uterine bleeding at the latter end of reproductive life with a normal-sized uterus. It is essential to rule out endometrial pathology by prior sampling. The availability of the levonorgestrel intrauterine system has reduced the demand for ablative techniques.

There is a range of different endometrial ablative techniques available with different risks, efficacies and costs. The first-generation techniques include transcervical resection of endometrium, endometrial laser ablation, and radiofrequency endometrial ablation. The second-generation techniques are many, the most common ones in use being endometrial balloon ablation and microwave endometrial ablation. The benefits with this procedure are avoiding the complications associated with hysterectomy and increased cost-effectiveness. It is a day-case procedure and the postoperative recovery is rapid.

The patient needs to be warned that her expectations, such as relief from dysmenorrhoea and premenstrual syndrome, may not be met. The menstrual blood loss may not alter or it may remain unacceptable, requiring further treatment. Amenorrhoea rates vary from 10 to 75%, and satisfaction rates from 55 to 90%. Pharmacological treatment of the endometrium before the procedure with gonadotrophin releasing hormone (GnRH) analogue or danazol improves the efficacy.

Patient information sheets should be given, along with verbal counselling, to include the individual operator's results in terms of satisfaction rates and menstrual outcome, including amenorrhoea rate and reoperation rate. The complications involved in the procedure (i.e. anaesthetic complications, perforation, a small risk of hysterectomy) should be discussed, depending upon the method being used. The need to continue contraception is emphasized. Advice should also be given that vaginal discharge is expected for up to 3 weeks and crampy pains for the first few days.

## Answer key and marking scheme

*A good candidate will discuss the indications, criteria to be fulfilled before the procedure, benefits, risks and points to discuss whilst counselling the patients.*

### Indications

Symptoms and signs such as anaemia, impairment of social and personal                 1 mark
life requires treatment.
Other alternatives of treatment, i.e. medical and progesterone intrauterine
system, must have been discussed or tried.

The technique is suitable for treatment of dysfunctional uterine bleeding at the       1 mark
latter end of reproductive life with a normal-sized uterus.

It is essential to rule out endometrial pathology by prior sampling.                   1 mark

### Techniques

There is a range of different endometrial ablative techniques available with           1 mark
different risks, efficacies and costs.
The first-generation techniques include transcervical resection of
endometrium, endometrial laser ablation, and radiofrequency endometrial
ablation.
The second-generation techniques are many, the most common ones in use
being endometrial balloon ablation and microwave endometrial ablation.

### Benefits

The benefits with this procedure are avoiding the complications associated             1 mark
with hysterectomy and increased cost-effectiveness.

It is a day-case procedure in most cases; occasionally, overnight stay for             1 mark
observation is required.

### Risks

The expectations of the patient such as relief from dysmenorrhoea and                  1 mark
premenstrual syndrome, may not be met.
The menstrual blood loss may not alter or may remain unacceptable requiring
further treatment.
Amenorrhoea rates vary from 10% to 75%, and satisfaction rates from 55% to
90%.

### Counselling

Patient information sheets should be given, along with verbal counselling covering the
following points:

- The individual operator's results, in terms of satisfaction                          1 mark
- Menstrual outcome, including amenorrhoea rate and reoperation rate

- Complications of the particular technique, including a small risk of      1 mark
  hysterectomy
- Treatment with danazol or GnRH analogues 6 weeks before treatment
  improves efficacy of the procedure. The need to continue contraception     1 mark
- Advice that vaginal discharge is expected for up to 3 weeks

## Suggested reading:

Scottish Intercollegiate Guidelines Network. *Hysteroscopic Surgery. A National Clinical Guideline.* SIGN publication no. 37. Edinburgh: SIGN; 1999 (**www.show.scot.nhs.uk/sign/home.htm**).

# **PAPER 2**: OBSTETRICS

1. Appraise the use of Doppler for fetus in the practice of obstetrics.

2. Discuss in brief how you would plan the strategy to reduce the rising caesarean section rate in your hospital. Justify your proposals.

3. A GP calls about a concerned woman who is 16 weeks pregnant and has been in contact with a child with varicella. Discuss the advice you will give regarding this episode.

4. How would you manage a primigravid woman at 37 weeks gestation with a breech presentation?

5. You see a para 2 during on-call hours at 34 weeks gestation complaining of fever with chills, vomiting and back pain for 2 days. She has had two such episodes prior to pregnancy. Dipstick of urine is positive for leucocyes and nitrites. Give the details of your plan of management.

1. Appraise in brief the use of Doppler for fetus in the practice of obstetrics.

*A good candidate will emphasize that use of Doppler is beneficial only in high-risk pregnancies, such as those affected by pre-eclampsia or intrauterine growth restriction. Mention the pros and cons associated with the use of Doppler.*

### Uses of Doppler
Doppler ultrasound provides a reliable method for auscultation and monitoring of fetal heart in late pregnancy and labour.                                   1 mark

It is a surrogate marker for placental vascular resistance, so it is useful to monitor pregnancies complicated by uteroplacental pathology.                   2 marks

Good correlation between absent or reversed end diastolic velocity in umbilical artery and perinatal mortality – 67% sensitivity and 98% specificity. Small-for-gestation (SGA) infants with elevated indices are three times more likely to be admitted in neonatal intensive care units.                        1 mark

### Pros
38% reduction in odds of fetal death.                                          1 mark

44% reduction in antenatal admissions.                                         1 mark
10% reduction in rate of interventions, such as induction of labour.
(*The figures for the events are not mandatory for writing*)

Some experts believe that Dopplers have the potential to aid the timing of delivery. Decisions are gestation dependent (GRIT, Growth Restriction Intervention Trial).                                                               1 mark

Colour-flow Doppler is useful in diagnosis of renal agenesis and cardiac anomaly in fetus.                                                              1 mark
Power Doppler sonography is better than colour Doppler sonography in prenatal diagnosis of fetal vascular anomalies.

### Cons
Doppler has been shown to be beneficial in high-risk pregnancy but not in low-risk pregnancy.                                                           1 mark

It cannot be used in isolation. The whole clinical scenario needs to be considered before clinical decision making.                                     1 mark

## Suggested reading

Kingdom JCP, Rodeck CH. Umbilical artery Doppler – more harm than good? *Br J Obstet Gynaecol* 1997; 104: 393–6.

Neilson JP, Alfirevic Z. Doppler ultrasound for fetal assessment in high risk pregnancies [systematic review] in The Cochrane Library, Issue 3, 2000. Oxford: Update software.

2. Discuss in brief how you would plan the strategy to reduce the rising caesarean section rate in your hospital. Justify your proposals.

*A good candidate will point out the important causes of rising caesarean sections and give practical measures to minimise the caesarean section rate. Don not forget to back this up with evidence base.*

Rising caesarean sections are giving concerns about increased maternal morbidity and mortality (*Why Mothers Die*). Set evidence based guidelines, protocols to ensure optimal outcome for both mother and baby. (*WHO Partogram Study*)

1 mark

Education of all staff involved in the management of parturient, greater input from senior staff on the delivery suite, multidisciplinary forum (*Good practice*).

1 mark

Regular audits for monitoring practice (*Clinical Governance*).

1 mark

**Evidence Base:**
Offering external cephalic version to women with uncomplicated singleton breech pregnanncy at term reduces the caesarean section rate done for this indication significantly (*RCOG guideline derived from randomised controlled trials*).

1 mark

Conducting trial of scar in women with previous caesarean section done for a non-recurrent indication is associated with 70% success of vaginal delivery (*observational studies*).

1 mark

Correct diagnosis of labour and correct physical representation of the data on cervicographs (*WHO Partogram Study*).

1 mark

Routine amniotomy should be discouraged as it does not improve outcome apart from reducing the duration of labour by up to 50 minutes but increases the incidence of cardiotocograph (CTG) artefacts (*UK Amniotomy trial*)

1 mark

30 minute increments in oxytocin infusion regimen to prevent uterine hyperstimulation and fetal hypoxia. 1:1 midwifery care and support of the mother with antenatal preparation and education. (*Towards safer childbirth*)

1 mark

Continuous CTG monitoring should not be routinely done in low risk labours.

1 mark

CTG abnormalities should prompt fetal blood sampling to establish true fetal acidosis (*NICE guideline*).

1 mark

## Suggested reading

Macfarlane A, Chamberlain G. What is happening to the caesarean section rates? *Lancet* 1993; 342: 1005–6.

Paul RH, Miller DA. Caesarean birth: how to reduce the rate. *Am J Obstet Gynecol* 1995; 172: 1903–7.

3. A GP calls about a concerned woman who is 16 weeks pregnant and has been in contact with a child with varicella. Discuss the advice you will give regarding this episode.

*A good candidate will know that the details of contact and previous history of chickenpox are important. Booking serum to be checked for varicella zoster IgG if any doubts of immunity; do not send the patient to the maternity hospital for this.*
*Reassure that most women are immune and most pregnancies are unharmed. If not immune, zoster immune globulin (ZIG) should be administered. Counsel regarding 2% risk of congenital varicella syndrome. Arrange for midtrimester anomaly scan.*

**History**
Ask about the details of contact history with particular respect to the certainty of the infection, the infectiousness, and the degree of exposure.  1 mark

The previous history of chickenpox in the woman is a reasonable indicator of her immunity.  1 mark

**Investigations**
If there is any doubt regarding the immune status, or if there has been contact (with no previous history of varicella), varicella zoster IgG titre should be checked.  1 mark

This can be arranged from the serum saved at booking. It is not advisable to bring the patient into hospital.  1 mark

Arrange for detailed ultrasound at 19–20 weeks to rule out anomalies.  1 mark

**Counselling**
Most women (85%) are immune and can be reassured.  1 mark

If the patient is not immune and develops primary varicella zoster infection or shows serological evidence of seroconversion, there is up to 2% risk of congenital varicella syndrome in the fetus.  1 mark

She then will need to be informed of the implications.  1 mark

Congenital varicella syndrome consists of skin scarring, limb hypoplasia, eye defects and neurological abnormalities.  1 mark

Give the patient zoster immune globulin (ZIG) 0.2–0.4 mg/kg if she is not immune.  1 mark

## Suggested reading:

RCOG. *Green Top Guideline No. 13: Chickenpox in Pregnancy.* London: RCOG Press, 1997.

4.  How would you manage a primigravid woman at 37 weeks gestation with a breech presentation?

---

*Discuss external cephalic version (ECV), vaginal breech delivery, and elective caesarean section, i.e. counsel mother regarding risks and benefits. amd allow informed choice. Elective caesarean section versus planned vaginal breech delivery: evidence in favour of caesarean section to reduce fetal morbidity and mortality.*

Confirm presentation by ultrasound and rule out placenta praevia, malformation.                                                                              1 mark
Also check for liquor volume, free cord and flexed head.

**External cephalic version**
All women with a breech presentation in an uncomplicated pregnancy at term should be offered external cephalic version (ECV).                                   1 mark

Performed on the labour ward; cardiotocography (CTG) before and after ECV; anti-D if Rhesus negative (Kleihauer).                                             1 mark

Pros: halves the rate of caesarean section done for breech presentation.
Cons: failure of procedure, possibility of emergency caesarean section if fetal distress develops (<1%).                                                          1 mark

Tocolysis is effective, both when used routinely or selectively                     1 mark

**Elective caesarean section**
Benefits: chance to turn spontaneously, decreased fetal respiratory morbidity if done beyond 39 weeks.                                                           1 mark

Reduced risks of neonatal morbidity and mortality, this is the safest mode of delivery for a baby in breech presentation.                                       1 mark

Risks: Thromboembolic events, haemorrhage and infection.                            1 mark
Risk of spontaneous breech labour is higher at a later gestation, leading in turn to a higher risk of emergency caesarean section (which is associated with higher morbidity as compared with elective caesarean section).

**Trial of vaginal delivery**
Higher risks of fetal morbidity and mortality (1.23% v. 0.09% for elective lower segment caesarean section, LSCS) and hence vaginal delivery is not favoured.       1 mark
Trial of labour is not offered in presence of medical or obstetric complications which are associated with mechanical obstruction to labour.

**Counselling** a patient includes description of vaginal breech delivery, 20% rate    1 mark
of failure ending in emergency LSCS, the need for trained personnel to be
present at delivery. She should also be informed that the likelihood of vaginal
delivery during next pregnancy after a caesarian section, is about 70%.

## Suggested reading:

Hofmeyr GJ, Hannah ME. Planned Caesarean section for term breech delivery
[Cochrane Review], in The Cochrane Library, Issue 3, 2000. Oxford: Update
software.

RCOG. *RCOG Guideline No. 20:The Management of Breech Presentation*: London:
RCOG Press; 2001.

5. You see a para 2 during on-call hours at 34 weeks gestation complaining of fever with chills, vomiting and back pain for 2 days. She has had two such episodes prior to pregnancy. Dipstick of urine is positive for leucocytes and nitrites. Give the details of your plan of management.

*A good candidate will structure the clinical approach into history, examination, investigations, treatment and follow-up.*

**History and examination**                                                    1 mark
Most likely diagnosis is pyelonephritis.

**Observations**
Temperature/pulse/blood pressure.

**Investigations**
Full blood count, serum urea, creatinine and electrolytes, urine and blood      1 mark
cultures.

If no clinical improvement, renal ultrasound scans in the first instance and    1 mark
plain X-ray abdomen if necessary, because the benefits outweigh any fetal risk
of radiation. Involvement of renal physician is desirable.
Acute pyelonephritis increases the risk of premature labour. Establishing fetal
well-being once maternal condition is stabilized is necessary.

**Supportive management**
Monitor vital signs frequently, including urine output.                         1 mark

Intravenous hydration to establish urine output of at least 30 ml/h.            1 mark

In case of severe complications of acute pyelonephritis, such as septic shock,  1 mark
adult respiratory distress syndrome, or chronic renal infection,
multidisciplinary approach with intensive care is required.
If urinary obstruction is diagnosed, urological input is required.

**Medical treatment**
Appropriate intravenous antimicrobial therapy whilst awaiting culture and       1 mark
sensitivities report. Penicillins and cephalosporins are usually the first choice,
although an aminoglycoside such as gentamicin may be required in the case of
septicaemia or resistant organisms in women allergic to both penicillin and
cephalosporin.

Repeat haematological and blood chemistry studies according to patient's        1 mark
condition.
Change to oral antibiotics when afebrile, and encourage oral fluid intake when
vomiting subsides.

**Follow-up**                                                                    1 mark
Discharge after patient has been afebrile for 24 h but continue antibiotics for
10–14 days.
Repeat urine culture 1-2 weeks after the antibiotic therapy is completed.        1 mark
Recurrent bacteruria warrants antibiotic treatment for the duration of
pregnancy.

## Suggested reading:

Vazquez JC, Villar J. Treatments for symptomatic urinary tract infections during
    pregnancy [Cochrane Review] in The Cochrane Library, Issue 3, 2000. Oxford:
    Update software.

# PAPER 2: GYNAECOLOGY

1. A 20-year-old woman is seen 2 days after an episode of sexual intercourse in which the condom split during coitus. Outline in brief how you will deal with this patient's request for contraception.

2. A 17-year-old girl is referred by her GP with a history of vaginal bleeding at 9 weeks gestation. Ultrasound reveals a molar pregnancy. Explore her further management.

3. A 57-year-old woman taking a cyclical hormone replacement for 1 year complains of irregular vaginal bleeding for 3 months. Her cervical smears have always been negative, and she is up to date with them. Her pelvic examination is normal. Discuss the choices of investigations for this patient.

4. A 45-year-old woman is scheduled to undergo hysterectomy for menor-rhagia. Discuss concurrent salpingo-oophorectomy.

5. 'Treatment with intracytoplasmic sperm injection (ICSI) should not be offered to all patients who need *in vitro* fertilization (IVF).' Debate this statement.

1. A 20-year-old woman is seen 2 days after an episode of sexual intercourse in which the condom split during coitus. Outline in brief how you will deal with this patient's request for contraception.

*A good candidate will take detailed history and rule out contraindications. Explain the methods available (PC4, Levonelle or intrauterine device), their risks, failure rates and the importance of follow-up. Advise that the next period may be early or late.*

### History and examination
Take detailed menstrual history, and timing of unprotected sexual intercourse in relation to the current cycle, history of recent pelvic infection, medical history (including migraine, and thromboembolism).     1 mark
Perform a pelvic examination if pregnancy is suspected (along with urine pregnancy test if history of previous unprotected intercourse) or before fitting coil.

### High-dose combined oral contraceptive pill (PC4)
If the patient has no contraindications, emergency combined pills or PC4 100 μg ethinyloestradiol with 250 μg levonorgestrel repeated in 12 h can be offered along with appropriate instructions.     1 mark

### Progesterone-only pills (Levonelle)
If the above history is positive, 0.75 mg levonorgestrel taken 12 h apart has equal efficacy.     1 mark

This is now the treatment of choice even without any past medical history because of the fewer side-effects as compared with high-dose combined pills.     1 mark

### Intrauterine device     1 mark
An intrauterine device (IUD) is an option as long as it is fitted within 5 days of earliest ovulation. Counsel, screen for infection, and fit copper IUD.

### Counselling
Explore the patient's attitude to possible failure of the regimen and continuation of the pregnancy.     1 mark
If pregnancy is suspected and diagnosed, it should be managed as for any other unintended pregnancy, i.e. termination of pregnancy is an option.

The practice of abstinence or careful use of the barrier method until the onset of the next menses should be advised.     1 mark

### Documentation
1 mark

Record the woman's decision to use emergency contraception after full discussion backed by the information leaflet.

### Future contraception
1 mark

Future contraception must be discussed in a sympathetic way and preferably arranged as appropriate.

### Follow-up
1 mark

The woman should be offered the opportunity to attend for follow-up within 3–4 weeks of the treatment, or earlier if she has any pain, bleeding or concerns. At follow-up, details of the post-treatment menstrual period should be recorded.

## Suggested reading:

Cheng L, Gülmezoglu AM, Ezcurra E, Van Look PFA. Interventions for emergency contraception [Cochrane Review], in The Cochrane Library, Issue 3, 2000. Oxford: Update software.

2. A 17-year-old girl is referred by her GP with a history of vaginal bleeding at 9 weeks gestation. Ultrasound reveals a molar pregnancy. Explore her further management.

*A good candidate will structure the answer to include investigations, suction-evacuation, obtain histopathology and register with one of the centres for further management and follow up. Anti-D for Rhesus-negative patients. Advice regarding future pregnancy and contraception should be mentioned.*

### Investigations
After explaining the condition to the patient, investigations such as full blood count, serum beta hCG, blood group and rhesus status are essential.                    1 mark

### Surgical treatment
Suction curettage is the method of choice.                                            1 mark
The products of conception should be sent for histopathological examination. Sound histopathology report is essential.

### Medical treatment
Medical termination of complete molar pregnancy, including cervical              1 mark
preparation before suction, should be avoided.
Withhold oxytocic infusions until completion of the procedure.

Anti-D is required if Rhesus negative.                                                 1 mark

### Supportive management
In the UK, there is an effective registration and treatment programme for        2 marks
gestational trophoblastic disease. After the confirmation of diagnosis by histopathology, the patient should be registered at one of the screening centres at London (Charing Cross), Sheffield or Dundee, from where further follow-up can be carried out.

If the symptoms persist after initial evacuation, consultation with the           1 mark
screening centre is sought before repeat evacuation.

The patient is advised not to become pregnant until after 6 months of normal     1 mark
human chorionic gonadotrophin (hCG) levels or until follow-up has been completed (whichever is earlier). Her risk of further molar pregnancy is 1 in 74.

Combined oral contraceptives are safe once hCG levels have returned to           1 mark
normal. Until then, use of any barrier method is desirable.

Urine and blood hCG levels are checked after 6 weeks of conclusion of any        1 mark
further pregnancies, to exclude recurrence.

## Suggested reading

RCOG. *RCOG Guideline No. 18: The Management of Gestational Trophoblastic Disease.* London: RCOG Press; 1999.

3. A 57-year-old woman taking a cyclical hormone replacement for 1 year complains of irregular vaginal bleeding for 3 months. Her cervical smears have always been negative, and she is up to date with them. Her pelvic examination is normal. Discuss the choices of investigations for this patient.

*A good candidate will explain the advantages and disadvantages of the options available: out-patient sonohysteroscopy, transvaginal scan, endometrial biopsy, out-patient saline hysterography, and inpatient hysteroscopy.*

The advantages and disadvantages of each method are explained to the patient.                    1 mark
Reassure the patient that most of the irregular vaginal bleeding is benign, but that it is important to rule out sinister pathology.

### In-patient investigations
Bimanual examination under anaesthesia, hysteroscopy with or without                             1 mark
endometrial biopsy.

This is suitable:                                                                                1 mark

- If facilities for out-patient investigations are not available
- For women with suspicious scan findings, recurrent bleeding or previous hyperplasia
- In women in whom out-patient hysteroscopy failed

### Out-patient endometrial biopsy (Pipelle, Vabra, Sharman curette)
Safe, reliable, cheap, easy to do.                                                               1 mark

May cause significant discomfort in 10%, of cases and there may be failure to                    1 mark
cannulate in 20% of cases. The pathology can be missed in some cases.

**Ultrasonography** (endometrial pathology and thickness, including the                          1 mark
visualization of the ovaries) is reliable, well tolerated, and will exclude the
need for histopathology in most cases. It is a useful investigation that provides
additional information.

The false positive rate is 10–20% and requires equipment and expertise.                          1 mark

### Out-patient sonohysteroscopy
Hysteroscopy has major diagnostic ability in terms of direct visualization of                    1 mark
pathology and directed endometrial biopsy. It is regarded as the gold standard
for diagnosis of postmenopausal bleeding.

Occasionally it may fail or be difficult, necessitating anaesthetic.                             1 mark

**Out-patient saline hysterosonography**

Pros: effective, easy procedure that can be done easily in clinic setting if an    1 mark
ultrasonography machine is available. Allows measurement of endometrial
thickness and outlines any irregularities in the endometrium, such as polyps
and fibroids.

Cons: histology is necessary for any suspicious findings; very rarely malignancy
may be missed.

## Suggested reading:

Ind T. Management of postmenopausal bleeding, in J Studd (ed.) *Progress in Obstetrics and Gynaecology*, 13. London: Churchill Livingstone; 1999. pp. 361–78.

Smith-Bindman R, Kerlikowske K, Feldstein VA *et al.* Endovaginal ultrasound to exclude endometrial cancer and other endometrial abnormalities. *JAMA* 1998, 280(17): 1510–17.

4. A 45-year-old woman is scheduled to undergo hysterectomy for menor-rhagia. Discuss concurrent salpingo-oophorectomy.

*A good candidate will discuss the benefits and risks of removing ovaries at hysterectomy and allow patient to make an informed choice.*

### Background for counselling
The average age at menopause is 51 years. Hysterectomy generally reduces this age limit by 2–3 years. This is further reduced by smoking and genetic reasons.    1 mark

Detailed history: smoking, family history of breast, bowel, ovarian cancer is important. Associated severe symptoms of premenstrual syndrome may help in the decision of oophorectomy.    1 mark

Pros of concurrent oophorectomy: relief from premenstrual syndrome, no possibility of residual ovary syndrome.    1 mark

Reduction of risk of ovarian cancer in future: reduces the risk 100-fold from a lifetime risk of 1%.    1 mark

Cons of concurrent oophorectomy: surgical menopause and its sequel.    1 mark

If done without adequate counselling and consent, this 'female castration' can result in great psychological morbidity.    1 mark

Need to take HRT for prolonged periods. This could have a potential for poor compliance.    1 mark

Oophorectomy does not reduce the risk of ovarian cancer completely because peritoneal metastases can still occur by metaplasia of coelomic tissue.    1 mark

### Risks associated with hormone replacement therapy    1 mark
Increased risk of breast cancer and venous thromboembolism associated with HRT: the risk of breast cancer increases from 2 in 1000 after 5 years to 7 in 1000 after 10 years of use. The risk for DVT increases from 11 in 100 000 for non-users to 27 in 100 000 for current users.

### Informed choice
After thorough counselling, the patient is allowed to make her own choice regarding having or not having concurrent oophorectomy.    1 mark

5. 'Treatment with intracytoplasmic sperm injection (ICSI) should not be offered to all patients who need *in vitro* fertilization (IVF).' Debate this statement.

*A good candidate should know that ICSI and IVF pregnancy rates are similar if semen parameters are normal. The benefit of ICSI is that fertilization rate is higher in patients who have sperm/egg interaction abnormalities, if semen quality is poor and in couples with IVF failures. The potential risks include that of higher risk of sex chromosomal abnormalities, higher demand on resources.*

### Advantages

The clinical pregnancy rate with ICSI per cycle is 26% while that with IVF is 15%.                                                                             1 mark

The fertilization rates for ICSI range between 33 and 70%.

The benefit of offering ICSI is that the 5% failure of fertilization rate will be reduced significantly for patients who have sperm/egg interaction abnormalities.                                                                       1 mark

Towards this end, couples with failed previous IVF should consider undergoing ICSI in future attempts because of the lower total fertilization failure.

ICSI is still preferred to using donor sperm by couples trying to conceive. Conceiving a child who is genetically their own appears to outweigh other considerations.                                                                       1 mark

### Potential disadvantages

*In vivo* protective mechanisms against abnormal sperm are bypassed.        1 mark
Possibly increased risk of abnormality, although it is too early to make definitive statements.

Increased sex chromosomal abnormalities in children born from ICSI: males more than females. There is postulation that the male offspring may have higher rates of subfertility due to some mutations in Y chromosome.          2 marks

ICSI is more costly and time consuming. It is also more invasive.           1 mark

### Rationale

There is evidence that when the semen analysis is normal, the fertilization rates per retrieved oocyte and pregnancy rates between ICSI and IVF are similar. Hence, ICSI should not be offered to all those who need IVF.        2 marks

### Candidates for ICSI

On balance, ICSI should be offered for:                                     1 mark

- Abnormal semen analysis: fewer than 1.5 million motile sperms or less than 5% normal forms recovered from ejaculate
- Poor or no fertilization in prior IVF cycle

## Suggested reading:

Van Rumste MME, Evers JLH, Farquhar CM, Blake DA. Intra-cytoplasmic sperm injection versus partial zona dissection, subzonal insemination and conventional techniques for oocyte insemination during *in vitro* fertilization [systematic review], in The Cochrane Library, Issue 2, 2000. Oxford: Update software.

# PAPER 3: OBSTETRICS

1. A multipara is admitted at 38 weeks with vulval herpetic lesions. She gives a history of herpes simplex in the last pregnancy. Justify your advice to this woman regarding her further management.

2. A primigravida has a mid-trimester scan at which the fetus is diagnosed to have congenital diaphragmatic hernia. Discuss the issues involved in the management of the pregnancy.

3. Critically evaluate the methods available for detecting diabetes mellitus in pregnancy and describe a practical model of screening in brief.

4. Whilst conducting a forceps delivery for delayed second stage, you encounter shoulder dystocia. What is the rationale of manoeuvres that you will attempt?

5. Critically comment on the need for antenatal beds in an obstetric unit and appraise the role of day assessment unit.

1. A multipara is admitted at 38 weeks with vulval herpetic lesions. She gives a history of herpes simplex in the last pregnancy. Justify your advice to this woman regarding her further management.

*A good candidate should give the rationale behind the antenatal management, choice of mode of delivery and postpartum care. Do not forget that full marks will not be allotted unless justification is given for each piece of advice.*

### Antenatal
The treatment should be in keeping with the patient's clinical condition. Recurrent attacks can be asymptomatic.                                         1 mark
Repeated viral cultures and swabs in late pregnancy are not useful in management.

**Supportive:** saline bathing and analgesia may be adequate in mild cases.      1 mark

### Medical treatment
It is appropriate to involve a genitourinary physician in discussion about the    1 mark
use of antiviral drugs and screening for sexually transmitted infection.

Acyclovir may be successful in suppressing the lesions at the onset of            1 mark
labour.

### Delivery
Vaginal delivery is appropriate in the absence of active lesions at the onset of  1 mark
labour.

### Surgical management
In the presence of active lesions in labour, there is evidence that the risks of   1 mark
vaginal delivery for the fetus are small and must be weighed against the risks
of caesarean section to the mother.

If the membranes have been ruptured for over 4 h when active lesions are          1 mark
present in the genital tract, vaginal delivery is appropriate as the rate of vertical
transmission rate is unaltered by caesarean section

With active infection, invasive monitoring with fetal scalp electrode and fetal    1 mark
blood sampling should not be used. These measures reduce the risk of vertical
transmission.

### Postnatal
The patient should be advised to report early signs of infection (e.g. lethargy,   1 mark
poor feeding or lesions) in the baby.
Breastfeeding is not contraindicated unless she has lesions on the breast.

Reassure that the risk of neonatal herpes is low in spite of the presence of active lesions, as this is not a primary infection.

1 mark

## Suggested reading:

Smith JR, Cowan FM, Munday P. Management of herpes simplex virus infection in pregnancy. *Br J Obstet Gynaecol* 1998; 105(3): 255–60.

2. A primigravida has a mid-trimester scan at which the fetus is diagnosed to have congenital diaphragmatic hernia. Discuss the issues involved in the management of the pregnancy.

*A good candidate will structure the approach of management into antenatal, intrapartum and postnatal periods. Presence of experienced neonatologist at birth is vital.*

### Antenatal

Congenital diaphragmatic hernia diagnosed before the twenth-fifth week of pregnancy carries 58% mortality.                                        1 mark

A detailed scan is organized to look for the extent of the defect (herniation of the liver and/or stomach into the chest, bilaterality are very poor prognostic factors) and other anomalies, such as cardiac anomalies especially ventricular septal defect and tetralogy of Fallot, pulmonary hypoplasia, genitourinary and skeletal anomalies.

Counselling and support for the parents is important.                  1 mark
Referral to a tertiary centre with expertise in fetal medicine is advisable.

Up to 20% of fetuses have chromosomal abnormalities. Hence, chromosomal     1 mark
analysis is offered via amniocentesis or cordocentesis.

If additional anomalies or defects are found, termination of pregnancy should   1 mark
be discussed.

Arrange for the parents to meet the paediatrician/paediatric surgeon who will   1 mark
explain the surgery involved as well as the prognosis.

Therapeutic thoracentesis has been used in the third trimester to improve fetal   1 mark
cardiovascular dynamics.
Successful *in utero* surgery has been described but has significant
complications, including preterm premature rupture of membranes, preterm
labour and fetal death.

Monitoring the pregnancy closely for development of polyhydramnios and its   1 mark
sequel is desirable.

### Delivery

Experienced paediatrician to be present at delivery to resuscitate the newborn.   1 mark
Ensure that delivery occurs in a unit where the services of paediatric surgeon
are available on hand.

The condition is not a contraindication for vaginal delivery.          1 mark

**Postnatal** 1 mark

Encourage expression of breast milk if mother wishes to breastfeed.

Reassure that the risk of recurrence is low (2–4%).

The outcome for either immediate (within 24 h of birth) or delayed (until stabilized) repair of congenital diaphragmatic hernia appears to be similar.

## Suggested reading:

Moyer V, Moya F, Tibboel R, Losty P, Nagaya M, Lally KP. Late versus early surgical correction for congenital diaphragmatic hernia in newborn infants [Cochrane Review], in The Cochrane Library. Issue 3, 2000. Oxford: Update software.

3. Critically evaluate the methods available for detecting diabetes mellitus in pregnancy and describe a practical model of screening in brief.

---

*A good candidate will discuss the various risk factors specificity and sensitivity of various potential diabetic features, and tests such as glycosuria, 1 h 50 g glucose challenge test, 2 h glucose tolerance test (GTT), and discuss a model.*

Identifying women susceptible to gestational diabetes is important to prevent perinatal mortality and to improve the outcomes for the mother and her child.

### History 2 marks
Family history – first degree relative (parent or sibling of the pregnant woman).
Diabetic of any type and impaired glucose tolerance (IGT) or gestational diabetes in previous pregnancy or older Asian women.
These are some of the potential diabetic features, which have a sensitivity of 50% and specificity of 66%.

### Other high risk factors 1 mark
Body mass index >30.
Polyhydramnios.
Past obstetric history of large-birth-weight infant (>4500 g).
Previous unexplained stillbirth, fetal macrosomia.

(½ *mark each for any four of the above points*)

### Screening tests
Testing for glycosuria at each antenatal visit has high sensitivity (90%) but low 1 mark specificity.

1 h 50 g glucose challenge test at a threshold value of 7.8 mmol/l has both high 1 mark sensitivity (59%) and high specificity (91%).

Measuring fasting plasma glucose is easier screening test. With a threshold 1 mark value of 4.8 mmol/l it yields a sensitivity of 81% and a specificity of 76%.

Random blood glucose level estimation is widely used, although it has low 1 mark sensitivity (40%).
The use of glycosylated haemoglobin estimation is not popular because of its low sensitivity.

### Diagnostic test
High-risk patients generally have GTT at 26 weeks. When risk factors develop 1 mark after 26 weeks, the GTT should be performed immediately.

**Proposed model**

In view of practicalities, the urine should be tested at each antenatal visit. Timed blood glucose estimation should be performed at booking and 28-week visits, and when glycosuria of 1+ or more is detected.                    1 mark

75 g 2 h glucose tolerance test should be performed if the timed blood glucose is >6 mmol/l in the fasting state or 2 h postprandial or if the blood glucose level is >7 mmol/l within 2 h of food in high-risk patients and those with abnormal screening tests.                    1 mark

## Suggested reading

Coustan DR. Screening and testing for gestational diabetes mellitus. *Obstet Gynecol Clin North Am* 1996; 23(1): 125–36.

Maresh M. Glucose intolerance in pregnancy. *PACE review no. 97/03*. London: RCOG Press; 1997.

4. Whilst conducting a forceps delivery for delayed second stage, you encounter shoulder dystocia. What is the rationale of manoeuvres that you will attempt?

*A good candidate will write the sequence of manoeuvres used. Do not forget that calling for help is important.*

The success and safety in managing shoulder dystocia depends on the experience of the practitioner and knowledge of labour ward protocols for this emergency.
Have the time noted and counted off when the problem is recognized.

1 mark

**Call for help** – senior experienced obstetrician and midwife, neonatologist, anaesthetist, etc. The senior obstetrician on scene takes charge.

1 mark

**Episiotomy** is done or extended to allow space to perform the manoeuvres. Explore manually behind the head and find out whether the posterior shoulder of the fetus is in the hollow of the sacrum.

1 mark

**McRobert's manoeuvre** – the exaggerated flexion of the maternal hips releases the anterior shoulder by causing cephalad rotation of the symphysis pubis.

1 mark

Careful constant **traction** on the fetal head for 30 s in downward and backward direction together with maternal pushing and **suprapubic pressure** by an assistant helps to force the anterior shoulder under the pubic arch.

1 mark

The next step is to attempt **rotation of fetal shoulders** in an oblique diameter. Delivery of the posterior arm first may be helpful.

1 mark

The **Wood's corkscrew manoeuvre** is attempted next. Two fingers in front of the posterior shoulder attempt to rotate it through 180 degrees. This brings the lower posterior shoulder anteriorly underneath the pubic symphysis from where it can easily be hooked out.

1 mark

If still unsuccessful in resolving the shoulder dystocia, the next thing to do is to try **extraction of posterior arm** by sliding a hand in the vagina behind the posterior shoulder and sweeping the posterior arm of the fetus across the chest keeping the arm flexed at the elbow. Grasp the hand and pull it and the arm along the fetal head delivering the posterior arm.

1 mark

If these measures fail and the baby is still alive, the following can be undertaken by an experienced operator: **cleidotomy**, or **symphysiotomy**.

1 mark

**Zavanelli's manoeuvre** in which the head is replaced back into the pelvis and caesarean section is carried out.

1 mark

If the fetus dies during the manoeuvres, an experienced operator may undertake destructive procedures.

## Suggested reading

Johnston FD, Myerscough PR. Shoulder dystocia. *Br J Obstet Gynaecol* 1998; 105(8): 811–15.

5. Critically comment on the need for antenatal beds in an obstetric unit and appraise the role of day assessment unit.

*A good candidate will mention categories best managed as in-patients, use of gynaecology wards for some disorders. Certain categories of patients, such as fetal growth restriction and premature rupture of membranes can be managed in the day assessment unit. Advantages and disadvantages of the day assessment unit should be discussed.*

### In-patient care

Most patients managed antenatally as in-patients can be cared for adequately in the home environment.    2 marks

Certain categories of patients have to be managed in hospital, e.g. acute life-threatening conditions such as haemorrhage – major degree of placenta praevia, abruptio placentae, unstable lie (risk of cord prolapse), severe pre-eclampsia, uncontrolled diabetes (conditions that require intensive surveillance).

(*½ mark each for any four of the above conditions*)

Hospitalization can bring about removal from disadvantageous environment, e.g. abuse. It enables monitoring of patient under controlled conditions, e.g. titration of drug doses.    1 mark

Use of gynaecology ward for some disorders is common, e.g. hyperemesis, mid-trimester bleeding; however this does not avoid use of a bed.    1 mark

Place of day assessment unit – allows performing out-patient biophysical profiles, cardiotocography and blood tests for the rapid and complete assessment of the maternal and fetal health.    1 mark

### Advantages    2 marks

Reduction in hospital admissions, in convenience and cost.
Provision of speedy assessment and management in response to the problems and risk factors identified in pregnancy, especially relevant now that more routine antenatal care is concentrated in the community.
Consistency of approach (due to protocols).
Audit of management strategies.

### Disadvantages    2 marks

Temptation to keep problems as out-patients when they should be in-patients (guidelines and protocols helpful in this respect).
Psychological costs of anxiety generated by intensive appraisal.
Improved medical outcome is not confirmed.
There is potential for increased responsibility on the community midwife and family doctor.
The geographical location of the unit in relation to the patient's home and the

domestic circumstances could make daily trips to the day unit disadvantageous.

Consequences such as financial implications to the patient and the hospital, patient compliance, and education of the general practitioner and midwife are some of the other issues involved.

1 mark

## Suggested reading

Soothill PW, Ajayi R, Campbell S, *et al*. Effect of a fetal surveillance unit on admission of antenatal patients to hospital. *BMJ* 1991; 303(6797): 269–71.

# PAPER 3: GYNAECOLOGY

1. A woman who wishes to have hormone replacement therapy (HRT) is referred by her GP to the menopause clinic. Her elder sister had calf vein thrombosis whilst on HRT. Justify your approach to this problem.

2. A 27-year-old woman requests a brand containing a third-generation progestogen for contraception. Justify your reasons for prescribing it for her.

3. A 34-year-old parous woman whose recent cervical smear is reported as showing atypical glandular cells suggestive of cervical glandular intraepithelial neoplasia (CGIN) is referred by her GP. Justify how you will manage this finding.

4. A 42-year-old woman whose smears have been normal in the past is referred for menorrhagia resistant to medical treatment. She asks about the benefits and risks of subtotal abdominal hysterectomy. How will you counsel her?

5. Which categories of patients are at risk of venous thromboembolism following surgery? Outline the preventive measures that you would adopt to reduce the occurrence of this condition.

1. A woman who wishes to have hormone replacement therapy (HRT) is referred by her GP to the menopause clinic. Her elder sister had calf vein thrombosis whilst on HRT. Justify your approach to this problem.

*Thrombophilia screening for the patient and her sister should be offered. If screen is negative, HRT can be prescribed provided the patient is counselled regarding the benefits versus risks. Transdermal therapy is recommended. In case high-risk defects are detected, management must be liaised with centres with expertise in thrombophilia. Prophylactic anticoagulation with warfarin is desirable with HRT in such a case. Alternative treatments for osteoporosis should be offered.*

Explore the reason for the request e.g. osteoporosis or other symptoms of menopause, as well as risk factors for osteoporosis – thyrotoxicosis, hyperparathyroidism, alcohol abuse, malabsorption syndrome, etc.                    1 mark

Attempt to establish whether the patient's sister's venous thrombosis was confirmed objectively. The clinical diagnosis of deep vein thrombosis (DVT) is unreliable and objective testing is essential.                    1 mark

The patient's sister should be screened for thrombophilic defects if possible. Selective screening for thrombophilia is offered to the patient herself. This includes testing for proteins C and S, anti-thrombin III, and factor V Leiden deficiency.                    1 mark

When no underlying thrombophilia is identified, then HRT can be prescribed, provided the risks versus benefits are considered.
The need to report promptly if any symptoms compatible with venous thromboembolism arise should be stressed.                    1 mark

Transdermal therapy may be recommended in this situation because of the fact that transdermal estrogens do not alter the coagulation factors.                    1 mark

In case high-risk defect such as type I anti-thrombin deficiency is found, and the patient still wishes to take the HRT, it must be with prophylactic anticoagulation with coumarins.
Monitoring can be a difficult problem. It is best handled by a centre with expertise in thrombophilia management.                    1 mark

With other thrombophilic defects, there is currently insufficient evidence to recommend complete avoidance of the HRT, and in most cases the benefits will outweigh the perceived risks.                    1 mark

A clear discussion of the potential excess risk should occur with the woman, and transdermal therapy is recommended. This is documented clearly in the records.                    1 mark

If the reason for request is to prevent osteoporosis, alternatives such as          1 mark
tibolone or bisphosphonates can be offered.

Advice regarding healthy lifestyle such as stopping smoking, reducing              1 mark
alcohol intake, and increasing exercise can be given, along with information
leaflets and names of support groups and organizations.

## Suggested reading:

Hormone replacement therapy and venous thromboembolism. *RCOG Guideline No. 19*. London: RCOG Press; 1999.

2. A 27-year-old woman requests a brand containing a third-generation progestogen for contraception. Justify your reasons for prescribing it for her.

*A good candidate will demonstrate understanding of the possible risks of third-generation contraceptive pills, the reason for request, and the patient's relevant history. After counselling the patient appropriately, the patient should be allowed to make an informed choice.*

### Rationale
The risks of deep vein thrombosis (DVT) in healthy, non-pregnant woman     1 mark
not taking any contraceptive pills is 5 in 100 000, while in pregnancy it is 60 in 100 000.

Third-generation pills containing desogestrel or gestodene have a slightly     1 mark
higher incidence of DVT: risk of 25 in 100 000 versus 15 in 100 000 for second-generation pills containing norethisterone or levonoregestrel.

The rate of fatality is 1 in 100 000, but the morbidity is much higher with     1 mark
third-generation pills.

But third-generation pills are associated with greater cardioprotection and less     1 mark
androgenic side-effects.

### Reason for request     1 mark
Has she had problems with other pills?
Does she need something less androgenic because she has acne or hirsutism?

### History
Are there any predisposing factors to DVT (obesity, smoking)?     1 mark

Does she have a personal or family history of thromboembolic disorder (i.e. is     1 mark
there a need for thrombophilia screen particularly activated protein C resistance)?
Thrombophilia screening detects 70% of cases and can give 30% false-negative results.

Factor V Leiden deficiency is associated with a high risk of DVT in combined     1 mark
oral contraceptive pill users (240 in 100 000).

Possibility of using norgestimate-containing pills, which are cardioprotective     1 mark
and less androgenic than second-generation combined oral contraceptive pills.
Their higher risk of DVT is not at present established.

### Counselling

Provided the patient understands the risks and does not have any medical          1 mark
contraindication (and this is recorded in notes), it should be a matter of
personal choice as to which type of oral contraceptive is taken.

## Suggested reading

Skegg D. Third generation oral contraceptives. *BMJ* 2000; 321: 190–1.

CSM and Medicines Control Agency *Current Problems in Pharmacovigilance.* June
1999; 25: 12.

3. A 34-year-old parous woman whose recent cervical smear is reported as showing atypical glandular cells suggestive of cervical glandular intraepithelial neoplasia (CGIN) is referred by her GP. Justify how you will manage this finding.

*A good candidate will demonstrate the understanding that natural history of cervical glandular intraepithelial neoplasia is uncertain and it generally co-exists with cervical squamous intraepithelial neoplasia. Structure the clinical approach into examination, histology, surgical treatment – conservative and radical. Follow-up is important.*

Cervical glandular intraepithelial neoplasia (CGIN) has an uncertain natural    1 mark
history. CGIN is underdiagnosed because of replacement of surface columnar cells by benign metaplastic or dysplastic cells.
The size of the lesion is generally small and co-existent squamous cervical intraepithelial neoplasia (CIN) reduces the cytological sensitivity for glandular disease.

### Examination
Urgent clinical and colposcopic assessment should be done in order to    1 mark
determine whether an overt potentially invasive lesion is visible.

Colposcopy helps to define the extent of the lesion, take directed biopsies and    1 mark
exclude vaginal intraepithelial neoplasia and vaginal adenosis.

### Investigations
Careful assessment of the transformation zone is important. If CIN is present,    1 mark
the transformation zone should be excised concurrently.

In cases of high-grade abnormality, endometrial sampling should be carried    1 mark
out along with colposcopy.

### Management
Cone biopsy more than 25 mm long with uninvolved cone margins is optimal    1 mark
management for CGIN.

Large loop excision of transformation zone (LLETZ) is an effective alternative    1 mark
for treatment.

If the margin of excision of the lesion is not clear or is involved, a repeat cone    1 mark
biopsy or a total hysterectomy should be considered, depending on the woman's desire to retain fertility, uterus and after understanding the need for follow-up in conservative management.

Follow-up cytology with Ayre's spatula and endocervical brush is essential.          1 mark

The cone biopsy may identify invasive adenocarcinoma, which then requires a          1 mark
radical hysterectomy if operable.

## Suggested reading

Cullimore JE, Luesley DM, Rollason TP, *et al.* A prospective study of conization of the
cervix in the management of cervical glandular intraepithelial neoplasia – a preliminary report. *Br J Obstet Gynaecol* 1992; 99: 314–18.

Kumar G, Howell R. Cervical glandular neoplasia [PACE article]. *The Obstetrician
and Gynaecologist* 2000; 1: 43–5

4. A 42-year-old woman whose smears have been normal in the past is referred for menorrhagia resistant to medical treatment. She asks about the benefits and risks of subtotal abdominal hysterectomy. How will you counsel her?

*A good candidate will discuss potential benefits and risks associated with subtotal hysterectomy. Advise that strong evidence is unavailable neither in favour of nor against the same. Provided that the patient understands the pros and cons, she can choose the type of hysterectomy that she wishes to have.*

**Potential benefits**

Shorter anaesthetic and operation time, translating into reduced morbidity.          1 mark

Reduced risk of primary haemorrhage and damage to the surrounding organs, such as the bladder and the ureterus.          1 mark

Less morbidity from secondary haemorrhage, haematoma, bladder and bowel dysfunction, infection, tubal prolapse and vault granulations.          1 mark

Potential of early resumption of sexual activity, lesser incidence of dyspareunia and sexual dysfunction with better vaginal lubrication.          1 mark

**Potential disadvantages**

Can menstruate from the endometrial remnants.          1 mark

Need to continue cervical smears.          1 mark

Cervical pathology such as chronic cervicitis causing discharge, polyps and stump carcinoma (up to 0.3%) can arise in the future after subtotal hysterectomy, which might necessitate further treatment.          1 mark

There is no substantial evidence available for or against the advantages of the subtotal hysterectomy.          1 mark

In view of normal smears in the past, the patient can be given the choice of total or subtotal hysterectomy provided she understands the pros and cons involved in both the procedures.          1 mark

Provide information leaflets and document the fact that the potential risks and benefits have been discussed with the patient.          1 mark

## Suggested reading

Thakar R, Mollison J, Manyonda IT. Total versus subtotal hysterectomy: the last great controversy in gynecological surgery? *Contemp Rev Obstet Gynecol* 1998: 61–5.

5. Which categories of patients are at risk of venous thromboembolism following surgery? Outline the preventive measures that you would adopt to reduce the occurrence of this condition.

*A good candidate will outline the pharmacological and non-pharmacological measures and the strategy should be based on the risk assessment of an individual patient and the extent of surgery.*

**High-risk** patients include those:                                    1 mark

- with three or more moderate risk factors
- undergoing major surgery for gynaecological cancer
- with a family history of venous thromboembolism (VTE), or suffering from paralysis or immobilization undergoing major surgery lasting over 30 min.

**Moderate risk factors** include:                                      3 marks

- minor surgery (<30 min) in patients with a personal or family history of thromboembolic disease or thrombophilia
- operations expected to last over 30 min
- extended laparoscopic surgery
- age over 40 years
- obesity (>80 kg)
- gross varicose veins
- current infection
- immobility before surgery for more than 4 days
- major concurrent disease, e.g. heart or lung disease, inflammatory bowel disease, nephrotic syndrome, non-gynaecological malignancy, heart failure or recent myocardial infarction
- combined oral contraceptive pill

(½ *mark each for any six of the above points*)

**Preoperative**
Adequate preoperative assessment of the patient (including plans to switch to      1 mark
heparin perioperatively in patients already on warfarin if appropriate).

Heparin prophylaxis should be used:
**Dose:** Unfractionated heparin (UH) 5000 iu subcutaneously 8-hourly.             1 mark
Low-molecular-weight heparin (e.g. enoxaparin 40 mg/day) – has advantage
of once-daily dosage, is as effective and probably safer than UH.

**Time and duration:** should be discussed (begin heparin 12 h before surgery       1 mark
given at a site away from the proposed wound and continue for 5 days or until
fully mobilized).

**Side-effects**: heparin prophylaxis is associated with thrombocytopoenia and an increased risk of bleeding (wound haematoma), but there are no significant changes in postoperative haemoglobin or blood transfusion requirements.

1 mark

**Intraoperative**
Thromboembolic deterrent stockings and/or calf compression/stimulation devices are recommended.

1 mark

**Postoperative**
Early mobilization and adequate hydration of the patient are desirable. Thromboembolic deterrent stockings.

1 mark

## Suggested reading

Macklon N, Greer I. Thromboprophylaxis in obstetrics and gynaecology. Personal Assessment in Continuing Education. *Review No. 95/10.* London: RCOG Press; 1995.

# PAPER 4: OBSTETRICS

1. A primigravida is admitted in early labour with spontaneous rupture of membranes at 42 weeks. The liquor is thick meconium stained. How does this influence your management?

2. A 20-year-old woman who is taking phenytoin sodium for grand mal epilepsy is keen on conception. Discuss the preconceptual, antenatal and postnatal care specific to her condition.

3. A 35-year-old primigravida has come to see you to discuss her screen-positive result for Down's syndrome, which is reported as 1 : 100. How will you counsel her?

4. You see a Jehovah's Witness (a religious sect that does not accept blood transfusions) in her third pregnancy at 12 weeks gestation in the booking clinic. What are the salient features in managing this patient?

5. A 28-year-old woman is referred by her GP with a history of previous three consecutive first-trimester miscarriages. Justify the investigations carried out for this condition in the prepregnancy clinic.

1. A primigravida is admitted in early labour with spontaneous rupture of membranes at 42 weeks. The liquor is thick meconium stained. How does this influence your management?

*A good candidate will know the risks associated with thick meconium stained amniotic fluid. Continuous fetal heart rate (FHR) monitoring, use of fetal blood sampling in case of abnormal FHR, indication for caesarean delivery and presence of neonatologist at delivery should be discussed.*

### Rationale
Meconium is relatively common in postmature pregnancy, and appears stale    1 mark
and dilute.
Passage of meconium is associated with an increased risk of intrapartum
stillbirth and neonatal death.

Various measures of morbidity, such as low Apgar scores or lowered acid–base    1 mark
status, are also corelated to thick meconium stained liquor.

Fresh, thick meconium reflects reduced amniotic fluid volume at the onset of    1 mark
labour, which in itself is a significant risk factor.
It may be a sign of impaired placental function, which exposes the fetus to risk
of hypoxia during labour and meconium aspiration syndrome at birth.

### Supportive management
If meconium is detected, continuous electronic fetal monitoring is    1 mark
recommended.
Amnioinfusion can be considered, although its value has not been established.

If fetal heart rate (FHR) remains normal, no specific action need be taken    1 mark
except to avoid actions such as supine position and acute epidural hypotension
that might precipitate acute hypoxia in the fetus.

### Medical management
If the labour is progressing well, it is appropriate to perform fetal scalp blood    1 mark
sampling (FBS) for unsatisfactory cardiotocography and allow labour to
continue if the results of pH and base excess are within normal limits. FBS
might have to repeated if the delivery is not imminent.

A neonatologist should be present at delivery.    1 mark

If the baby is alert at birth, there is no further need to do anything else.    1 mark
Although there is no evidence in support of routine suction of the pharynx as
soon as possible after delivery, it is probably acceptable as long as it is gentle,
because it can, at times, precipitate meconium aspiration.

**Surgical treatment**

If the FHR pattern becomes abnormal in early labour (<4–5 cm), caesarean    1 mark
section is a better option.

This decision is also influenced by the presence of other factors, such as    1 mark
postmaturity, intrauterine growth restriction, and maternal wishes.

## Suggested reading

Steer PJ, Danielian PJ. Fetal distress in labor in DK James, PJ Steer, CP Weiner , and
B Gonik (eds). *High Risk Pregnancy Management Options*, 2nd edn. London:
WB Saunders; 1999. pp. 1089–94.

2. A 20-year-old woman who is taking phenytoin sodium for grand mal epilepsy is keen on conception. Discuss the preconceptual, antenatal and postnatal care specific to her condition.

*A good candidate will structure the answer according to preconceptual, antenatal and postpartum care.*

### Prenatal

Phenytoin in periconceptual period increases the risks of congenital heart defects, orofacial clefts and other minor malformations.                1 mark

Risk to fetus from the fit is small but significant.                              1 mark.
Reassure that most women have uneventful pregnancies with healthy neonate.

Rate of congenital malformation is 2.5% in non-epileptic women and 6.5% in epileptics on medication. The risk of congenital malformations increases with polytherapy.                1 mark
Control of epilepsy should be optimized before pregnancy.
If fit-free for many years, consider stopping the medication. This should be a fully informed decision after counselling, especially the risk of losing driving licence in the event of a seizure.                1 mark

The woman should be advised to take folic acid 5 mg daily for at least 12 weeks before pregnancy. This should be continued throughout pregnancy.                1 mark

### Antenatal

Care shared with neurologist.                                                  1 mark
Offer prenatal screening with maternal serum alpha fetoprotein and detailed high-resolution scan at 18–20 weeks, including cardiac scan at 22 weeks.

Growth scans if poorly controlled epileptic.                                   1 mark
Vitamin K 20 mg daily for the last 4 weeks of pregnancy.

In most cases, the frequency of fits is not altered by pregnancy. Measuring drug levels and adjusting dose of antiepileptics is not required if the patient is fit-free.                1 mark
Also, advice regarding avoidance of stress and ensuring adequate sleep is helpful.

### Postnatal

Vitamin K for the neonate.                                                     1 mark
No contraindication to breastfeeding.

If dose of anticonvulsant was increased specifically due to pregnancy, it would be reduced in puerperium.      1 mark

Contraception with high-dose oestrogen pills is desirable. Higher doses of progesterone-only pill is also required due to the enzyme-inducing activity of phenytoin.

## Suggested reading

Scottish Obstetric Guidelines and Audit Project. *The Management of Pregnancy In Women with Epilepsy. A Clinical Practice Guideline for Professionals Involved in Maternity Care.* Scottish Obstetric Guidelines and Audit Project: **www.show.scot.nhs.uk/sign/sogap1.htm**.

3. A 35-year-old primigravida has come to see you to discuss her screen-positive result for Down's syndrome, which is reported as 1 : 100. How will you counsel her?

---

*Check gestational age. Explain what screen-positive and screen-negative result means. Diagnostic test i.e. karyotyping by amniocentesis or fetal blood sampling, is advised. The parents are informed that the options, in case Down's syndrome is confirmed, will be termination of pregnancy or expectant management.*

After introduction and explaining to the woman the reason for this visit, her booking ultrasound scan is reviewed to check the gestational age and the final expected due date.

*1 mark*

### What is Down's syndrome?

*1 mark*

The chromosomal defect where there is trisomy 21. There is no treatment. Explain the features and prognosis for Down's syndrome. It is variable, but it is associated with mental retardation, besides various other systems being involved.

### Interpretation of result

Screen-positive does not mean that the fetus has Down's syndrome. It only means that the woman's risk is increased from the age-related risk of 1 in 350 to 1 in 100 in this case.

*1 mark*

Similarly, a screen-negative test means that the risk of Down's syndrome is low with a 30% false-negative rate.

*1 mark*

### Confirmatory tests

For confirmatory diagnosis, karyotyping by amniocentesis/fetal blood sampling is recommended.

*1 mark*

The procedure and possible risks and complications (including that of miscarriage of about 1 in 150) need to be explained. An information leaflet is given to the patient along with support and more counselling if required

*1 mark*

### Management

If Down's syndrome is confirmed, the parents can be offered termination of pregnancy. The procedure involved is explained to the woman and her partner. Intracardiac potassium chloride is recommended over 21 weeks so that the baby is not born alive.

*1 mark*

The other option of expectant management and its implications in terms of long-term care required should be explained clearly.

*1 mark*

The names and addresses of support groups such as SATFA (Support

*1 mark*

Around Termination for Fetal Abnormality), should be offered.
Explain the possibility of earlier prenatal diagnosis in her next pregnancy and
referral for genetic counselling.

**Recurrence risk**
The risk of Down's syndrome at the age of 35 years is 1 in 350. The woman's       1 mark
risk of this recurring is 0.43% plus age-specific risk for non-disjunction, and
10% plus age-specific risk in case of translocation.

4. You see a Jehovah's witness (a religious sect that does not accept blood transfusions) in her third pregnancy at 12 weeks gestation in the booking clinic. What are the salient features in managing this patient?

*Patient's decision to decline blood transfusion is to be respected. Booking should be done in a unit with all the facilities for prompt management of haemorrhage including hysterectomy. Measures to minimize harm from haemorrhage should form the substance of the answer.*

### Antenatal
The woman's religious beliefs and likeliness for refusal for blood transfusion should be recorded in the notes. The detailed documentation of what is acceptable (blood products, plasma etc.) is essential. The woman and her partner should be offered the chance to read and discuss the treatment guidelines of the unit. — 1 mark

She should advised that if massive haemorrhage occurs, there is increased risk that hysterectomy will be required. — 1 mark

If she decides against blood transfusion in any circumstances, she should be booked for delivery in a unit with all the facilities for prompt management of haemorrhage, including hysterectomy. — 1 mark

The woman's blood group and antibody status should be checked in the usual way, and haemoglobin should be checked regularly. Haematinics should be given throughout the pregnancy. — 1 mark

An ultrasound scan for placental position should be arranged. — 1 mark

If any complications are noted during the antenatal period, or when the patient is admitted in labour, the consultant obstetrician must be informed. If caesarean section is required a consultant obstetrician should carry it out. — 1 mark

### Delivery
Experienced staff should manage the labour routinely. Uterotonics should be given in the third stage. — 1 mark

The principal of management of haemorrhage in this woman would be to avoid delay and have low threshold for intervention. — 1 mark
Consultant anaesthetist and haematologist should be involved early.
Intravenous crystalloid and Haemaccel should be used for volume expansion.

The woman must be kept informed and the staff must maintain professional attitude at all times. — 1 mark
Autotransfusion is an option but is limited by mother's haemoglobin.

**Postnatal**

When the mother is discharged from the hospital, she should be advised to      1 mark
report promptly if she has any concerns about bleeding in puerperium.

## Suggested reading

Lewis G, Drife, J. *Report on Confidential Enquiries into Maternal Deaths in the UK 1991–1993*. London: HMSO; 1998. pp. 44–5.

5. A 28-year-old woman is referred by her GP with a history of previous three consecutive first-trimester miscarriages. Justify the investigations carried out for this condition in the prepregnancy clinic.

*A good candidate will know the reasons behind doing the following investigations in patients with recurrent miscarriage: parental karyotyping, pelvic ultrasound, midfollicular LH/FSH, antiphospholipid antibodies, thrombophilia screen, and high vaginal swab. The candidate will also know that renal, liver and thyroid function tests, as well as $HbA_{1c}$ and TORCH screens, are not performed routinely.*

Loss of consecutive three confirmed pregnancies is termed as recurrent miscarriage. Detailed history is taken of the gestation at previous losses, menstrual pattern and medical history.

### Investigations offered to all patients

Parental karyotyping detects chromosomal abnormality found in up to 3–5% of patients.    1 mark

Pelvic ultrasound enables visualization of polycystic ovaries.    1 mark
Occasionally, it is also helpful in detecting uterine abnormalities such as bicornuate and subseptate uterus.

Midfollicular LH/FSH detects hypersecretion of LH, as in polycystic ovaries    1 mark
and premature menopause.

15% of women with recurrent first-trimester losses, and 30% of women with    2 marks
second-trimester miscarriages, may have antiphospholipid (APL) antibodies,
which may be the causative factor in the recurrent miscarriage. At present,
two separate measurements 6 weeks apart of a prolonged dRVVT (dilute
Russel viper venom test) and/or raised anticardiolipin antibody (IgG/IgM)
is diagnostic.

20% of these women have thrombophilic defects. Treatment with low-dose    2 marks
aspirin and heparin has showed improved outcome. Hence it is worthwhile
screening for thrombophilia: activated protein C resistance (APCR), proteins
C and S, factor XIII and anti-thrombin III deficiency.

Women who are positive for bacterial vaginosis in first or early second    1 mark
trimester have a increased risk of late second-trimester miscarriage. As this
condition is easily detectable and treatable, high vaginal swab is done in order
to screen and treat these women.

**Selective investigations**
Thyroid function tests, liver function tests and renal function tests are done if          1 mark
clinically indicated.
Laparoscopy and hysteroscopy are required to confirm urogenital anomalies
when they are suspected. A select group with anomalies may benefit from
cervical cerclage.

Glucose tolerance test, TORCH screen (to detect antibodies against          1 mark
toxoplasmosis, cytomegalovirus, herpes) and human leucocyte antigen have
no value in the investigation of recurrent miscarriages.

## Suggested reading

Li TC. Guide for practitioners: recurrent miscarriage principles of management. *Hum Reprod* 1998; 13: 478–82.

Rai R, Reagan L. Recurrent miscarriage. *CME Self-Assessment Test Review 96/08.* London: RCOG Press; 1996.

# PAPER 4: GYNAECOLOGY

1. A 34-year-old patient becomes pregnant spontaneously after many years of primary infertility. At referral to the antenatal clinic, it is reported that her most recent cervical cytology shows severe dyskaryosis. Justify the alternatives in her management.

2. Discuss the pros and cons of different tests to assess tubal patency in infertility.

3. A 47-year-old woman who still menstruates has been commenced on hormone replacement therapy (HRT). Advise her regarding contraception.

4. A 33-year-old woman is referred by her GP with severe symptoms of pre-menstrual syndrome. She has tried different over-the-counter medications. Discuss the options in the management of this patient.

5. Discuss the steps a laparoscopic surgeon can take to minimize bowel damage, and describe briefly the management of bowel injury at laparoscopy.

1. A 34-year-old patient becomes pregnant spontaneously after many years of primary infertility . At referral to the antenatal clinic, it is reported that her most recent cervical cytology shows severe dyskaryosis. Justify the alternatives in her management.

*The candidate should know the natural history of cervical intraepithelial neoplasia (CIN), need for colposcopy, the correlation between cytology and invasion, biopsy if invasion is suspected, possible/perceived complications, and the alternative of serial colposcopy with possible risks.*

**Natural history**

In the natural history of cervical intraepithelial neoplasia (CIN), only about 30% of CIN III will develop invasion in the next 20 years.       1 mark

The relationship between cytology, colposcopic findings and histology is not accurate.       1 mark

**Investigations**

The patient is seen, counselled and has colposcopic evaluation within 4 weeks of referral. Reassure the patient that colposcopy will not harm the fetus or cause miscarriage.       1 mark

Colposcopic impression correlates with the histopathology in approximately 85% of cases. It is essential to visualize whole transformation zone, as a small field of CIN may be present within the much wider areas of metaplasia.       1 mark

**Surgical Management**

For the grossly visible cervical lesion, biopsy (large loop excision of transformation zone, LLETZ) is the norm.       1 mark

**Advantages of LLETZ**

Unlike the cone biopsy, this is not associated with major morbidity such as haemorrhage, infection or miscarriage. Diagnosis and treatment can be done concurrently.       1 mark

If there is suspicion of invasion, wedge biopsy of the most abnormal area of cervix is also acceptable.       1 mark
Punch biopsies are unreliable in diagnosis of invasive disease. Besides, there is a higher risk of haemorrhage and unsatisfactory sample in pregnancy.

**Conservative management (alternative option)**

Regular colposcopic examination (every 6–8 weeks) without biopsy throughout pregnancy if the lesion does not look suspicious of invasion.       1 mark

The lesion is treated postpartum. It is advisable that this should be reserved for the expert colposcopist.

1 mark

### Counselling

Counsel the patient – explain the advantages and risks of both the alternatives, and manage according to her choice.

1 mark

## Suggested reading

Luesley DM. Difficult situations and management problems, in: DM Luesley, MI Shafi and JA Jordan. *Handbook of Colposcopy*, 1st edn. London: Chapman & Hall; 1996. pp. 110–12.

2. Discuss the pros and cons of different tests to assess tubal patency in infertility.

*A good candidate will discuss the advantages and disadvantages associated with laparoscopic dye test, hysterosalpingogram, contrast sonosalpingography and fallopioscopy.*

**Laparoscopic chromopertubation** is considered to be the gold standard.
Pros: simultaneous assessment of other pelvic pathology, such as peritubal adhesions and endometriosis, is possible.

1 mark

Concomitant procedures, such as salpingoscopy, hysteroscopy, adhesiolysis or tubal reconstructive surgery, can be performed. There is no exposure to radiation.

1 mark

Cons: risk of anaesthesia; potential risks and complications of laparoscopy, exact site of obstruction can be difficult to determine.

1 mark

**Hysterosalpingogram (HSG)**
Pros: cheap, simple out-patient procedure without need for anaesthesia. Uterine cavity can be assessed with exact site of tubal block. Therapeutic effect is controversial and is seen more with oil-based dye than water-based dye (pregnancy rates are doubled following oil-soluble dye HSG).

1 mark

Cons: exposure to radiation and pain; no information is gained on pelvic pathology; high false-positive rate (85% sensitivity and specificity as compared to Lap and dye test); pelvic infection in less than 1%.

1 mark

**Hysterosalpingo-contrast-sonography (HyCoSy)**
Pros: office procedure allowing dynamic assessment of the pelvis; no anaesthetic or radiation exposure. No anaphylactic reaction as no iodine contrast dye involved; less expensive and painful. The sensitivity and specificity is comparable to HSG.

1 mark

Cons: requirement of personnel trained in transvaginal scanning; inability to assess accurately peritubal adhesions and pelvic pathology.

1 mark

**Methylene blue test, gas hydrotubation**
Simple, low-tech procedures without exposure to radiation or anaesthesia. The disadvantage is that differentiation between unilateral and bilateral patency is impossible. Culdocentesis needs to be performed correctly.

1 mark

**Selective salpingography and fallopioscopy**
Pros: enables better selection of candidates who will benefit from tubal surgery. Treatment can be done at the same time by balloon tuboplasty. Advantages include avoidance of general anaesthesia, surgery and expensive hospitalization.

1 mark

Cons: requires expertise, training and time.                    1 mark

## Suggested reading

Watson AJS, Maguiness SD. Diagnostic and therapeutic aspects of tubal patency testing, in: J Studd (ed.) *Progress in Obstetrics and Gynaecology*, 13. London: Churchill
Livingstone; 1999. pp. 297–310.

3. A 47-year-old woman who still menstruates regularly has been commenced on hormone replacement therapy (HRT). Advise her regarding
contraception.

*HRT is not a contraceptive. The types of contraception she can use need to be discussed along
with advice about the duration they should be continued.*

### Necessity for contraception
HRT is not contraceptive – the dose of oestrogen within the HRT does not            1 mark
reliably suppress ovulation.

If a woman commences HRT before her periods cease, she must be advised to           1 mark
use contraception as her natural menopause will be masked by HRT-induced
bleeds.

### When to stop contraception
Advise her to stop HRT and measure FSH level approximately after 6 weeks            1 mark
and 4–8 weeks thereafter.
If the two FSH levels are above 30 mU/ml, it suggests significant loss of
ovarian function.
Contraception can be discontinued after one further year after that date
beyond age of 50 years or two further years under 50 years.

If menstruation returns or FSH level is in the normal reproductive age group        1 mark
range, contraception should be continued.

In a woman unwilling to temporarily stop HRT, advise continuation of                1 mark
contraception until the age of 55 years when it can be assumed that natural
fertility has been completely lost.

### Which contraceptive method?
Barrier methods such as condoms and diaphragms are quite effective in this          1 mark
age group.
Progesterone-only pill can be taken in conjunction with HRT and is widely
prescribed.

The administration of depot medroxyprogesterone acetate and norethisterone          1 mark
enanthate may cause amenorrhoea in up to 35% of patients, which may cause
anxiety about pregnancy or onset of menopause.

If an intrauterine device is *in situ*, it can be removed at 55 years. The bleeding  1 mark
pattern should be monitored carefully.

The levonorgestrel intrauterine system (LNG-IUS, Mirena) can be ideal for            1 mark
menorrhagia where pathology is ruled out. It can be a contraceptive and

progesterone arm of the HRT at the same time, along with being therapeutic for heavy bleeds.

Women who have sexual intercourse infrequently may practise coitus interruptus and postcoital contraception.

1 mark

Female sterilization or vasectomy of partner are the irreversible methods of contraception.
Natural family planning methods could be difficult in those with irregular periods, though it has obvious advantages in this age group because of declining fertility and coital rates.

## Suggested reading

Whitehead M, Godfree V. Contraception, in *Hormone Replacement Therapy – Your Questions Answered*, 1st edn. Edinburgh: Churchill Livingstone; 1996. pp. 213–21.

4. A 33-year-old woman is referred by her GP with severe symptoms of premenstrual syndrome (PMS). She has tried different over-the-counter
medications. Discuss the options in the management of this patient.

*A good candidate will follow the format of history, examination, investigations (PMS diary,
psychological evaluation of patients with noncyclical symptoms) and treatment options –
non-pharmacological, pharmacological (non-hormonal and hormonal) and surgery.*

**History**                                                                1 mark
Take history – personal, social, menstrual symptoms. The aim of this is to
measure the severity of cyclical symptoms, the degree of underlying
psychological dysfunction, and the degree of disruption of the patient's life.

**Investigation**                                                          1 mark
Ask her to keep symptom diary for 2 months and review before diagnosing
PMS. This will enable differentiating PMS from non-menstrual-related
disorders.

**Supportive treatment**
Explain the condition (education and counselling). It might be reassuring for    1 mark
her to know that a lot of women have some form of PMS.
Rest, isolation, music therapy, diet manipulation, self-help groups,
acupuncture, stress management.

**Medical (non-hormonal ) treatment**                                      1 mark
Pyridoxine, essential fatty acids, vitamins, zinc, diuretics, nonsteroidal anti-
inflammatory drugs, antidepressants, selective serotonin reuptake inhibitors
(e.g. fluoxetine).
(*allot 1 mark for mentioning any four of the above medications*)

If the woman has continuous, noncyclical psychological problems wrongly       1 mark
attributed to the PMS, psychological evaluation and treatment is warranted.

**Hormonal treatment**                                                     2 marks
Progestogens, oral contraceptive pills, danazol, bromocriptine, hormone
implants, continuous oestrogen with levonorgestrel intrauterine system
(Mirena) can be tried.

**Surgical treatment**
If everything else fails and patient wants bilateral oophorectomy, the various
issues that need to be discussed are:

- **Gonadotrophin releasing hormone (GnRH) analogues** – as a            1 mark
  diagnostic tool to assess whether bilateral oophorectomy will achieve the
  necessary symptom control.

- **Risks of premature menopause** – explanation involves description of the    1 mark
  symptoms of menopause; the need for long-term HRT    postoperatively
  and the associated risks
- **The type of surgical procedure** – the risks and complications involved in    1 mark
  hysterectomy with bilateral salpingo-oophorectomy

## Suggested reading

O'Brien S, Chenoy R. Premenstrual syndrome, in: RW Shaw, PW Soutter, and SL
    Stanton,( eds). *Gynaecology*, 2nd edn. London: Churchill Livingstone; 1997 pp.
    359–71.

5. Discuss the steps a laparoscopic surgeon can take to minimize bowel damage, and describe briefly the management of bowel injury at laparoscopy.

*A good candidate will structure the answer into pre- and intraoperative strategies to prevent bowel injury. In case of recognized injury, seeking help from a surgeon is necessary. Postoperative low threshold of suspicion and appropriate management will be secondary and tertiary preventive measures.*

### Preoperative
Adequate training in operative techniques, including directing instruments appropriately, helps reduce the rate of injuries.                                                 1 mark

Recognize the cases in which the risk of damage is increased, such as previous abdominal surgery carried out for bowel disease or previous abdominal sepsis.                1 mark

### Intraoperative
Open laparoscopy: the risk to normally situated bowel may be reduced by Hasson technique.                                                                               1 mark

Using an alternative site of entry: the initial trocar may be placed away from the site of previous incision in an attempt to avoid fixed bowel.                            1 mark
Insertion of a microlaparoscope in the left upper quadrant with the subsequent insertion of the umbilical trocar under direct vision reduces the risk in adherent bowel.

After insertion, veress needle should be checked for correct intraperitoneal position by Palmer's test and noting pressure at entry.                                         1 mark
Creation of high-pressure pneumoperitoneum reduces initial trocar injury. This high-pressure setting is then lowered as soon as safe abdominal entry is confirmed.

The use of guarded point instruments and the introduction of second and subsequent ports under direct vision may reduce the risk further in all patients.                    1 mark

The recognition of injury at the time of operation may be assisted by noting the contents of bowel on the tip of instruments. It may go unnoticed if the injured area is empty or not in the field of vision.                                              1 mark

Minor injury to the bowel may be repaired laparoscopically by a surgeon or gynaecologist experienced in laparoscopic suturing. Second opinion from surgeon is helpful in uncertain cases.                                                         1 mark

In most cases, it is safer to perform a laparotomy (usually with a midline    1 mark
vertical incision) to allow careful inspection of the whole bowel and open
repair of any damage.

**Postoperative**
Postoperatively, bowel injury should be considered in the presence of excessive    1 mark
pain, tachycardia, pyrexia or peritonitis. High index of suspicion and early
opinion from a surgeon is essential to avoid further complications and
mortality.

## Suggested reading

A consensus document concerning laparoscopic entry techniques, *Gynaecol Endosc*
1999; 8: 403–6.

# PAPER 5: OBSTETRICS

1. Discuss the place of vaginal delivery in a woman with a history of caesarean section in previous pregnancy.

2. A waitress in a school canteen is 8 weeks pregnant and wishes to know which infections that she might acquire as a result of her job and which might harm her fetus. How will you counsel her?

3. A primigravida with no past medical history is seen in the antenatal clinic at 33 weeks gestation with severe pruritus. She is found to have abnormal liver function tests and raised bile acids. Hepatitis serology is negative. Justify the principles of management.

4. A 33-year-old multipara, who is in the thirty-ninth week of an uncomplicated pregnancy, requests induction of labour. What issues will you counsel her on?

5. Critically evaluate the statement, 'Mortality from erythroblastosis fetalis should be anecdotal in the present age.'

1. Discuss the place of vaginal delivery in a woman with a history of caesarean section in previous pregnancy.

*A good candidate will discuss the benefits, indications and contraindications for vaginal birth as well as patient preference.*

**Prognosis**
Success rates for vaginal birth after caesarean section (VBAC) range from 60    1 mark
to 80%.
The likelihood of vaginal birth is altered by the indication for the first
caesarean section (including 'failure to progress').

**Pros**
The potential benefits of a successful trial of scar include – lesser material    1 mark
morbidity and mortality.

Fewer requirements for analgesia, shorter hospital stay.    1 mark

**Cons**
Possibility of increased risk of morbidity due to emergency caesarean section    1 mark
(CS), and ill effects of vaginal delivery on the pelvic floor (bowel and stress
incontinence, prolapse).

A previous classical CS or unknown uterine incision is a contraindication to    1 mark
VBAC (risk of rupture of scar of classical CS is four times more than scar of
lower segment caesarean section in a subsequent pregnancy and labour).

There is some evidence that the risks and benefits of VBAC for patients with an    1 mark
existing multiple pregnancy or breech presentation appear similar.

There is no place for home delivery in a woman who has had a caesarean    1 mark
section.

**Management issues**
In labour, presence of intravenous access, continuous monitoring and care    1 mark
under obstetrician are desirable.

The appropriate use of oxytocics for induction and augmentation of labour is    1 mark
acceptable and requires the same precautions that should always attend the use
of oxytocic agents. CESDI report point out that prostaglandin for induction of
labour in women with previous scar can increase risk of scar dehiscence.

Epidural analgesia is not contraindicated.    1 mark
The patient must be involved in the decision making (patient choice).

## Suggested reading

Enkin M, Keirse MJNC, Renfrew M, Neilson J. Labour and delivery after previous caesarean section, in *Guide to Effective Care in Pregnancy and Childbirth*, 2nd edn. Oxford: Oxford University Press; 1998. p. 284–93.

2. A waitress in the school canteen is 8 weeks pregnant and wishes to know which infections she might acquire as a result of her job and which might harm her fetus. How will you counsel her?

*A good candidate will discuss the mode of transmission of each infection, its sequel in pregnancy on the fetus and the steps to avoid it. The following infections should be discussed: transmissible from children: chickenpox, parvovirus B19, rubella, and cytomegalovirus (CMV); and food-borne infections, such as toxoplasmosis and listerosis.*

### Infections that could be transmitted from children

**Chickenpox**: if previous history of chickenpox is certain, then she can be reassured. If history is uncertain, advise to stay away from work environment until varicella zoster immunoglobulin titre is checked on the serum. If negative, she should consider changing job to one that does not involve contact with children, or she should stay at home.                      1 mark

If she is susceptible and is infected in the first trimester, there is 2% risk of congenital varicella syndrome (affects skin, limbs and eyes, and can cause psychomotor retardation).                                              1 mark

**Parvovirus B19**: if a pregnant woman who is not immune to this infection is affected, it can cause hydrops, anaemia or miscarriage.                 1 mark

Her immune status can be checked. If she is not immune, it is advisable to stay away from the work environment.                                          1 mark
In the event of fetal anaemia due to this infection, fetal blood transfusion may be required.

**Rubella**: immune status will be checked and if found to be susceptible, she is advised to discontinue work. It is strongly recommended to get vaccinated postpartum.                                                           1 mark

The risk of congenital rubella syndrome is highest in the first trimester, when it can lead to ocular, hearing and heart defects, and mental retardation. There is some risk after first trimester (<5%).                              1 mark

**Cytomegalovirus**: can affect in all trimesters, causing microcephaly, chorioretinitis, jaundice, hepatosplenomegaly and thrombocytopoenia in the newborn. Hearing loss and mental retardation can be delayed manifestations. Positive serology, however, does not confer full protection, and careful handling of body fluids (as it is acquired from infected urine and saliva) is recommended.                                                          1 mark
(*½ mark each for fetal effects and preventive step*)

**Food-borne infections**
**Listeriosis**: in mother, this can cause a flu-like febrile illness. It may cause mid-       1 mark
trimester miscarriage, preterm labour and perinatal listeriosis.

Careful attention to food hygiene can decrease the incidence of food-borne       1 mark
gastrointestinal infection.
The pregnant woman is advised to avoid  high-risk foods, such as soft cheese,
pate and raw vegetables stored in cool environment after preparation, e.g.
coleslaw.

**Toxoplasmosis**: to avoid toxoplasmosis, it is advisable to avoid ingestion of un-       1 mark
cooked/undercooked or cured meat and unwashed vegetables, and to stay
away from cats and sheep.

3. A primigravida, with no past medical history is seen in the antenatal clinic at 33 weeks gestation with severe pruritus. She is found to have abnormal liver function tests and raised bile acids. Hepatitis serology is negative. Justify the principles of management.

---

*A good candidate will mention history, examination and investigations as usual. Supportive, medical and surgical treatment and the reasons behind this management plan should be written. Allot ½ mark for each point mentioned in investigations and treatment.*

**History and examination** to rule out other disorders.                          1 mark
The most probable diagnosis in this case is intrahepatic cholestasis of pregnancy (ICP).
It is a diagnosis of exclusion.

**Antenatally**
**Investigations**
Other causes of cholestasis, such as gallstones, should be excluded with         1 mark
ultrasound.
Liver function tests, including prothrombin time, and bile acids should be checked regularly (twice weekly) to decide the optimum timing for delivery.

**Prognosis**
Once the diagnosis of ICP is made, the mother should be counselled about the     2 marks
possible risks to the fetus, such as spontaneous preterm delivery, intrapartum fetal distress and intrauterine death. There are some uncertainties surrounding the optimal way to manage this condition.

**Supportive management**
Close surveillance of the fetus can be done by a combination of daily            2 marks
cardiotocography, ultrasound scans for fetal growth every fortnight and for liquor volume and Doppler-blood flow analysis twice a week. It is not clear which parameter predicts accurately the risk of fetal death.

**Medical treatment**
Vitamin K (10 mg daily orally) given to the mother reduces the risk of           1 mark
maternal and fetal bleeding.
Vitamin K should be administered immediately postpartum to the baby to reduce the risk of intracranial bleeding.

Antihistamine such as terfenadine or chlorpheniramine may help relieve the       1 mark
pruritus.
Ursodeoxycholic acid is a choleretic agent and reduces serum bile acids, although it is not licensed for use in pregnancy.
A course of steroids must be given if delivery before 36 weeks is anticipated.

**Delivery/surgical management**

Active management with induction of labour at 37–38 weeks may be considered in view of the risk of perinatal mortality.

1 mark

Caesarean section is reserved for obstetric indications and fetal compromise.

**Postnatal**

Complete recovery is usual following delivery.

1 mark

The woman should be counselled that the risk of recurrence in future pregnancies is at least 50%. She should also be advised to avoid oral contraceptives containing oestrogen.

## Suggested reading

Davidson KM. Intrahepatic cholestasis of pregnancy. *Semin Perinatol* 1998; 22(2): 104–11.

4. A 33-year-old multipara, who is in the thirty-ninth week of an uncomplicated pregnancy, requests induction of labour. What issues will you counsel her on?

*A candidate should explain the risks and benefits of induction, management options and allow the patient to make an informed choice.*

Explore the reason for the woman's request, e. g. extreme discomfort due to diastasis of symphyseal joint. — 1 mark

There could be a valid domestic/social reason. — 1 mark

Past obstetric history is important, i.e. normal vaginal deliveries in the past or complicated deliveries after induction of labour. — 1 mark

### Alternative
Discuss the alternative of continuation of the pregnancy as this carries less risk if the fetal growth and well-being are satisfactory. — 1 mark

Bishop's score assessment is of critical importance. If the cervix is unfavourable, the need for induction of labour (IOL) should be reconsidered. — 1 mark

### Induction of labour
Explain the methods of induction and their possible adverse effects. The methods include PGE2 (vaginal/intracervical) and artificial rupture of membranes with or without intravenous oxytocin infusion. — 1 mark

### Complications of IOL
Discuss the risk of uterine hypertonia and intrapartum fetal distress, increased requirement of analgesia, prolongation of labour, increased risk of postpartum haemorrhage. — 1 mark

Possibly increased risk of operative interventions, i.e. forceps, caesarean section, fetal blood sampling. — 1 mark

Should induction fail, however, it should be explained beforehand that the risks of caesarean delivery outweigh any possible social benefits. In such an event, continuation of pregnancy may be an option. — 1 mark

### Informed decision
After full discussion, induction of labour may be justified according to the particular circumstances involved and any decision should be taken on an individual basis after informing the woman fully of any potential disadvantages. — 1 mark

## Suggested reading

Alfirevic Z, Howarth G, Gaussmann A. Oral misoprostol for induction of labour with a viable fetus [systematic review], Cochrane Pregnancy and Childbirth Group, in: The Cochrane Library, Issue 3, 2000. Oxford: Update software.

ROCG. Induction of labour. *Guideline No. 16.* London:  RCOG Press; 1998.

5.  Critically evaluate the statement, 'Mortality from erythroblastosis fetalis should be anecdotal in the present age.'

---

*A good candidate should exhibit the knowledge of the reasons behind sensitization, the reasons for the reduced incidence, and strategies for prevention of this problem.*

**Anti-D**

Administration of D immunoglobulin to the mother prevents the initial response that causes Rh immunization in 97% of cases. This has made the occurrence of the disease a relatively rare event.                                1 mark

**Reasons for decrease in incidence**                                   2 marks

The fall in the perinatal mortality and morbidity from this disorder has also been influenced by factors such as:

*   Small family size
*   Improved antenatal surveillance and intrauterine transfusion of the affected fetus
*   Early planned delivery with steroid cover if necessary
*   Improved neonatal intensive care
    (*allot ½ mark for each point mentioned*)

**Reasons for persistence**

There is still some low but persistent incidence of Rhesus immunization episodes due to omitted or failed prophylaxis and silent fetomaternal haemorrhage (FMH).                                                        1 mark

Three per cent of erythroblastosis is caused by immunization against other fetal antigenic groups such as C, c, E, e, K, k and M which is not preventable.    1 mark

**Strategies to minimize Rh sensitization**

Routine use of antenatal prophylaxis at 28 and 34 weeks.                 1 mark

Rigorous administration of anti-D to all Rhesus-negative women after potentially sensitizing procedures or incidents, such as spontaneous or induced abortions, chorionic villous sampling, amniocentesis, ectopic pregnancies, attempted external cephalic version, abdominal trauma, any form of uterine bleeding.                                                  2 marks
(*allot 2 marks for mentioning any four of the above* )

Use of appropriate dose of anti-D titrated by Kleihauer test, 250 IU before 20 weeks and 500 IU after 20 weeks gestation. Kleihauer test identifies FMH over 4 ml in 1.5% of patients who require extra anti-D.                         1 mark

Anti-D should be given any time up to 4 weeks after delivery to an Rh-      1 mark
negative mother with an Rh-positive baby, or a baby whose Rh D status cannot
be determined. The maximal protective effect is obtained if it administered
within 72 h of delivery.

## Suggested reading

Crowther C, Middleton P. Anti-D administration after childbirth for preventing
    Rhesus alloimmunisation [systematic review], Cochrane Pregnancy and
    Childbirth Group, in: The Cochrane Library, Issue 3, 2000. Oxford: Update
    software.

Whitfield CR. Rhesus disease: success but unfinished business, in PMS O'Brien (ed.)
    *The Yearbook of Obstetrics and Gynaecology*, Vol. 8. London: RCOG Press; 2000.
    pp. 161–80.

# PAPER 5: GYNAECOLOGY

1. A 32-year-old nulliparous woman presents with intermenstrual bleeding and occasional postcoital bleeding. She is found to have a 0.5-cm lesion on the cervix. The biopsy of this lesion confirms squamous carcinoma of cervix. How would you counsel this woman?

2. A couple who have been trying for a pregnancy for over 16 months are investigated for infertility and a diagnosis of unexplained infertility, is reached. Both are 27 years old and wish to know further options of management. How will you advise them?

3. A 28-year-old woman presented with a history of 6 weeks amenorrhoea and lower abdominal pain. Transvaginal ultrasound scan confirmed heterotopic twin pregnancy. Discuss the different options of management.

4. Discuss the medicolegal issues involved in female sterilization.

5. What are the pros and cons of the surgeries done for vault prolapse?

1. A 32-year-old nulliparous woman presents with intermenstrual bleeding and occasional postcoital bleeding. She is found to have a 0.5-cm lesion on the cervix. The biopsy of this lesion confirms squamous carcinoma of cervix. How would you counsel this woman?

*A good candidate will explain the diagnosis, further investigations, treatment options, and success rates and their potential risks and offer support and information leaflets.*

Explanation of diagnosis and further investigations should be given. Her options for treatment are discussed and brief idea of postoperative follow-up is given.  `1 mark`
The information is backed up by information leaflets and contacts of support groups.

**Investigations**
**Radiological**: intravenous urogram, chest X-ray.  `1 mark`
Other investigations that may be performed include computer-assisted homography (CT) scan and magnet resonance imaging (MRI) (to exclude parametrial and lymph node involvement).

Examination under anaesthesia is an essential step in determining the extent of the disease and in deciding optimum method of therapy.  `1 mark`
Cystoscopy is done at the same time.

**Treatment options**
Surgery: radical hysterectomy and pelvic lymphadenectomy together are often preferred in younger patient with lower-volume disease.  `1 mark`

The complications include those of anaesthesia and extensive surgery, such as haemorrhage and urinary problems (fistulae, infection, atonic bladder).  `1 mark`

Discuss ovarian conservation in surgery.  `1 mark`

Fertility-preserving surgery such as radical trachelectomy following a negative retroperitoneal lymphadenectomy is experimental.  `1 mark`

Radiotherapy is another option, although not preferred for young and fit women.It may be needed post-surgery if lymph nodes are positive for spread of the disease.  `1 mark`

Side effects include vaginal stenosis, infertility, ovarian failure and gastrointestinal disturbance.  `1 mark`

**Long-term follow-up**  `1 mark`
Survival after treatment: 95% 5-year survival.
Follow-up at regular intervals until disease free for 5 years.

## Suggested reading

American Cancer Society
http://www3.cancer.org/cancerinfo/load_cont.asp?st=tr&ct=8.

2. A couple who have been trying for a pregnancy for over 16 months are investigated for infertility, and a diagnosis of unexplained infertility is reached. Both are 27 years old and wish to know further options of management. How will you advise them?

---

*The management options as usual are do nothing, medical, surgical and supportive management. It is useful to mention which treatments are not useful.*

## Supportive
Advice regarding healthy lifestyle (stop smoking and reduce alcohol intake)     1 mark
and folic acid.
Timed intercourse is not helpful.

The couple should be informed of the various options of treatment and     1 mark
allowed to make an informed choice.
They should be given information leaflets to support the verbal counselling.

## Do nothing
The available evidence suggests that there is little to be gained by commencing     1 mark
treatment in unexplained infertility before the couples have been trying for
3 years.

About 40–65% of the couples will become pregnant within 3 years of this     1 mark
diagnosis without treatment.

## Medical
Ovulation induction with clomiphene citrate (CC) is empirical. One should     1 mark
remember its side effects, and association of its prolonged use (>12 months)
with ovarian tumours.
A trial for CC for six cycles is appropriate only in experimental setting.

Superovulation (gonadotrophin injections) with intrauterine insemination     1 mark
could be tried for three to four cycles.

With this approach, the monthly chance of conception is about 20%, the     1 mark
4-month cumulative conception rate is 40%, and the risk of twins is about
20%.

## Surgical
Gamete intrafallopian transfer (GIFT) may have a possible but unproved     1 mark
benefit.
The main disadvantage that has made it fall out of favour is need for
laparoscopy and more complicated ovarian stimulation protocol.

*In vitro* fertilization (IVF) is less invasive than GIFT and enables the study of       1 mark
fertilization and the selection of good-quality embryos before transfer into the
uterus.
It also avoids the need for laparoscopy and general anaesthesia.

Intracytoplasmic sperm injection is the final step offered in assisted conception       1 mark
if the fertilization is poor in IVF.

## Suggested reading

RCOG. The management of infertility in secondary care. *Evidence-Based Clinical
Guidelines No. 3*. London: RCOG Press; 1998.

3. A 28-year-old woman presented with a history of 6 weeks amenorrhoea and lower abdominal pain. Transvaginal ultrasound scan confirmed heterotopic twin pregnancy. Discuss the different options of management.

*A good candidate will discuss pros, cons, indications of laparoscopy versus laparotomy, salpingectomy versus salpingotomy, injection into sac under laparoscopic or ultrasonic guidance. Methotrexate is not an option.*

Heterotopic pregnancy is the occurrence of simultaneous intra- and extrauterine pregnancy.
**Laparoscopic treatment** is desirable for an ectopic pregnancy in a stable patient.

**Pros**                                                                          2 marks
Less blood loss, lower analgesic requirements, shorter hospital stay, quicker postoperative recovery time, and comparable intrauterine pregnancy (IUP) rates.
(½ *mark each for any four of the above points*)

**Cons**
Higher rate of persistent trophoblastic tissue after laparoscopic salpingotomy,        1 mark
requires training and equipment and is contraindicated in a shocked patient.
(½ *mark each for any two of the above points*).

**Laparotomy indications** are haemodynamic unstability, history of              1 mark
cardiovascular or respiratory problems, extensive pelvic adhesions.

**Pros**
Less expertise and equipment required, and it may be slightly quicker.           1 mark

**Cons**
Longer hospital stay, increased analgesic requirements, increased morbidity; in  2 marks
most cases laparoscopy would precede laparotomy for confirmation of the diagnosis.

**Salpingotomy versus salpingectomy**
Salpingectomy is to be preferred to salpingotomy when the contralateral tube      1 mark
is healthy.

Salpingotomy is reasonable if there is only one tube present. The patient is      1 mark
counselled that the incidence of repeat ectopic pregnancy in this situation is 20%.

**Local injection** of potassium chloride into the gestation sac either at        1 mark
laparoscopy or under ultrasound guidance is not an option because of concurrent intrauterine live pregnancy. Methotrexate is not advisable for the same reason.

Administration of anti-D if patient is Rhesus negative and not sensitized.

## Suggested reading

Hajenius PJ, Mol BWJ *et al.* Interventions for tubal ectopic pregancy [Cochrane review], in: The Cochrane Library, Issue 3, 2000. Oxford: Update software.

RCOG. The management of tubal pregnancies. *Guideline No. 21.* London: RCOG Press; 1999.

4. Discuss the medicolegal issues involved in female sterilization.

*A good candidate will discuss the negligence at various steps and strategies to minimize the risks. Preoperative counselling and consent, pregnancy test before the procedure. Intraoperative: incorrect technique or correct technique followed by recanalization, other complications. Postoperative: failure of procedure, migration of clips.*

Litigation in relation to female sterilization can be due to various reasons, such as failure of recognition by the surgeon that the patient was already pregnant at the time of the procedure. If the procedure is performed in the luteal phase of the menstrual cycle, there is a possibility that the patient is already pregnant.                                                   1 mark

Caution: perform a sensitive urine pregnancy test on every patient before the procedure.                                                                    1 mark
The patient should be explained that she herself is responsible for any pregnancy, that could have been conceived before the operation.

Failure of appropriate counselling, and therefore the failure to take appropriate informed consent, is an important cause for litigation                       1 mark

There is obligation on the part of the doctor to include in the discussion and document the following:                                                        2 marks

- Irreversibility of the procedure
- Alternative methods of contraception (vasectomy, coil)
- Risk of failure ( 1 in 200 procedures)
- Risk of ectopic pregnancy in case of failure
- Risk of visceral injury, laparotomy, anaesthetic

Inadvertent injury during access to, or while occluding, the tubes, such as application of clip accidentally to bowel, or thermal injury to bowel while using cautery.                                                                    1 mark

Open laparoscopy is designed to reduce the risk of visceral injury. Mechanical methods of sterilization eliminate the risks of thermal injuries. Performing the procedure under local anaesthesia eliminates the risks associated with general anaesthesia.                                            1 mark

The patient should be counselled appropriately regarding contraception to be used and if necessary continued until the next menstrual cycle after the procedure.                                                                     1 mark

Failure of operation either because of inadequate technique leading to continued tubal patency or correct technique followed by recanalization or fistula.                                                                        1 mark

**128**

The Bolam test is used to decide whether negligence has occurred.

Migration of clips following a normal application is a potential cause for
litigation. Migrated clip rarely causes morbidity, and reassurance is all that is
warranted.
Open fallen clips should be removed.

1 mark

## Suggested reading

Filshie GM. Sterilisation. *The Obstetrician and Gynaecologist* 1999; 1(1): 26–31.

5. What are the pros and cons of the surgeries done for vault prolapse?

---

*Comment on the principle advantages and disadvantages and success rates of each procedure, i.e. pelvic floor repair, sacrospinous ligament fixation, abdominal sacrocolpopexy, laparoscopic colposuspension, combined abdominovaginal procedure, and others.*

### Vaginal procedures
Posterior colporrhaphy causes shortening and narrowing of the vagina, which    1 mark
may cause dyspareunia.
Benefits: simpler procedure, relatively short postoperative recovery.

### Sacrospinous ligament fixation
Though it can be done bilaterally, fixing one side of the vagina to the    1 mark
sacrospinous ligament can suffice. It has 80–92% success rate.

Complications: damage to pudendal nerves and vessels, sciatic nerve, infection,    1 mark
dyspareunia, chronic perineal pain and failure.

Benefits: prevention of laparotomy, concurrent repair of cystocoele and    1 mark
rectocoele possible, reduced operation time and postoperative pain and
quicker recovery.

**Colpocleisis** (Le Fort's operation) can be done in old patients, even under    1 mark
local anaesthesia.
Risks: recurrent prolapse; stress incontinence exists with this procedure as well
as the fact that sexual intercourse is not possible.

High dissection of enterocoele and plication of uterosacral ligaments with    1 mark
their attachment to vaginal vault for support carries the risks of injury to
bowel and ureters with 10–15% risk of stress incontinence.

### Abdominal procedures
**Sling operation**: vaginal vault apices are attached to rectus sheath, which
changes the anatomy.
**Sacrocolpopexy**: retroperitoneal funnelling of sling from sacrum to vaginal    1 mark
vault. Advantage: high success rate (93–98%), associated with slightly longer
functional length of vagina.

Disadvantage: haemorrhage from presacral vessels, morbidity associated with    1 mark
laparotomy and infrequently the graft has to be removed due to infection or
erosion into the vagina or bowel. Stress incontinence may occur in 7–33% of
patients.

### Combined abdominoperineal procedure             1 mark
Zacharin's procedure: more anatomical repair, 93.5% success rate.

Disadvantage: requires more time and two surgeons.

**Laparoscopic sling procedure**                                    1 mark
Laparoscopic sacrocolpopexy: all the advantages of minimal access surgery and potential risk of failure of the procedure and risks inherent to laparoscopic surgery.
Long-term success rates not yet available.
(*allot ½ mark each for mentioning any of the two points mentioned in the above sections*)

## Suggested reading

Hobson PT, Boos K, Cardozo L. Management of vaginal vault prolapse. *Br J Obstet Gynaecol* 1998; 105: 13–17

# PAPER 6: OBSTETRICS

1. Debate the various options for delivery in a woman with prolonged second stage of labour due to occipito-posterior position of the fetal head below the spines with normal power and passage.

2. A multiparous patient at term is referred to the consultant clinic from community because of suspicion of a large baby. Justify your clinical approach in managing this patient.

3. Debate the use of nuchal fold translucency versus serum screening as the methods of antenatal screening for aneuploidy.

4. Discuss the prognosis and management of a twin pregnancy complicated by antenatal demise of one of the fetuses diagnosed at 30 weeks gestation.

5. A primigravida attends at 38 weeks with confirmed spontaneous rupture of membranes and a singleton fetus in cephalic presentation. She is not in labour and has been well thus far. Critically evaluate your options of managing this patient.

1. Debate the various options for delivery in a woman with prolonged second stage of labour due to occipito-posterior position of the fetal head below the spines with normal power and passage.

*Consider the various delivery options with their associated advantages and disadvantages: manual rotation and forceps, non-rotational forceps with face-to-pubis delivery, ventouse, lower segment caesarean section (LSCS), rotational forceps.*

Manual rotation to occipito-anterior position and delivery with forceps: risk of cord prolapse, adequate analgesia required.                            1 mark

Occipito-posterior delivery with non-rotational forceps: increased risk of third-degree perineal tear.                                              1 mark

**Ventouse delivery**, preferably by using Bird's occipito-posterior metal cup.    1 mark

Pros: lower risk of maternal injury, less analgesia required.                  1 mark

Cons: increased risk of failure (especially with silastic cup), risk of subgaleal haematoma and retinal haemorrhage in neonate.                          1 mark

**Caesarean section**                                                            1 mark
Pros: decreased fetal trauma.
Cons: increased maternal morbidity.

**Rotational forceps (Kielland's forceps)**
Pros: can avoid the morbidity associated with emergency caesarean section,     1 mark
shorter hospital stay, fewer failure rates compared with ventouse, higher satisfaction rate if patient expected to have vaginal delivery.

Cons: requires skill, experience, adequate analgesia, can cause spiral vaginal   2 marks
tears and other complications.

After assessing the woman and giving her appropriate information and advice,    1 mark
informed consent is essential whatever procedure is carried out.

## Suggested reading

Pearl ML, Roberts JM, Laros RK, Hurd WW. Vaginal delivery from the persistent occiput posterior position: influence on maternal and neonatal morbidity. *J Reprod Med* 1993; 38(12): 955–61.

Riethmuller D, Teffaud O, Eyraud JL, Sautiere JL, *et al.* Maternal and fetal prognosis of occipito-posterior presentation. *J Gynecol Obstet Biol Reprod (Paris)* 1999; 28(1): 41–7.

2. A multiparous patient at term is referred to the consultant clinic from community because of suspicion of a large baby. Justify your clinical approach in managing this patient.

---

*A good candidate will elicit history, perform examination, arrange for relevant investigations, and discuss supportive, medical and surgical management*

### Verification of the suspicion
**History** of weights of previous babies and details of previous deliveries     1 mark
(difficult or prolonged labours, perineal trauma, previous shoulder dystocia).
Predisposing factors: multiparity, postmaturity, diabetes.

**Clinical examination** for symphysiofundal height, polyhydramnios,     1 mark
engagement of presenting part.

### Investigations
Ultrasound (USS) for abdominal and head circumference and estimated fetal     1 mark
weight (EFW).
Carries error of ±15–20%, and is not an accurate predictor of large baby
and degree of difficulty in vaginal delivery.

USS also helps to rule out or confirm fetal anomaly, multiple gestation and     1 mark
polyhydramnios also rules out mistaken finding in large/obese mother.
Diabetes screen if necessary by random blood sugar or glucose tolerance test.

### Justification for caution/prognosis
Risks of macrosomia are higher risk of shoulder dystocia and perineal trauma     1 mark
in the form of third- or fourth-degree perineal tear.

### Supportive
If no macrosomia, treat as normal and reassure.     1 mark
If glucose tolerance test is impaired, dietary advice is in order. However, strict
control of blood sugar has not shown improved outcome. Presence of a
neonatologist at delivery and to observe the neonate for development of
hypoglycaemia is necessary.

### Medical
There is no alteration of risk of maternal or neonatal morbidity with     1 mark
induction of labour for suspected fetal macrosomia in non-diabetic women.
Management of gestational diabetes is done in conjunction with a physician
in a joint clinic. Insulin is commenced and titrated according to the blood
sugar levels.

Allow spontaneous onset of labour: normal cervicometric progress is not a     1 mark
safeguard.

Be prepared for shoulder dystocia: drills/protocols/experienced staff to be present at delivery.

1 mark

**Surgical**

Caesarean section can be offered taking the whole clinical situation into consideration and if the patient so wishes.
It carries the risk of increased maternal morbidity (relatively reduced neonatal morbidity).

1 mark

## Suggested reading

Irion O, Boulvain M. Induction of labour for suspected fetal macrosomia [Cochrane Review], in: The Cochrane Library, Issue 3, 2000. Oxford: Update software.

3. Debate the use of nuchal fold translucency versus serum screening as the methods of antenatal screening for aneuploidy.

*A good candidate should know the WHO criteria for the ideal screening test. The pros and cons of the two tests in terms of timing, detection rate, resources, etc. should be discussed.*

Timing: nuchal fold translucency (NFT), 12–14 weeks; serum screening, 15–18 weeks. Both are carried out to screen for Down's syndrome.　　1 mark

### Pros of NFT
Termination of pregnancy (TOP) if opted may be medically and psychologically easier in early rather than later gestation.　　1 mark
Earlier reassurance to the groups at risk.

Detection rate of anomalies is 80% for NFT (combined with serum testing and age).　　1 mark

Some preliminary trials using combination of maternal age, fetal nuchal translucency thickness, and maternal serum free beta-hCG and pregnancy-associated placental protein A (PAPPA) have shown that the detection of trisomy 21 in pregnancy at 10–14 weeks can be improved by up to 89% with a false-positive rate of 5%.　　1 mark

NFT may detect other conditions, e.g. cardiac anomalies.　　1 mark.
NFT is superior for multiple gestation where serum screening is not of value.

### Cons of NFT
May be illusory: earlier testing may detect some cases, that would eventually miscarry.　　1 mark

NFT is more costly in terms of resources of skill and time.　　1 mark
Reproducibility is questionable out of tertiary referral centres.

### Pros of serum screening
Widely offered in most centres in the UK, so experience of use is wide.　　1 mark
Easy to reproduce, as it is based on biochemical markers with little inter- or intraobserver variation.
Well-known test.

### Cons of serum screening
Detection rate, 60% with 5% false-positive rate.　　1 mark

Relatively late screening and late TOP.　　1 mark
Affected by different characteristics of the patient, such as obesity, diabetes and ethnicity; request forms have to be filled correctly to enable correction for these variables.

4. Discuss the prognosis and management of a twin pregnancy complicated by antenatal demise of one of the fetuses diagnosed at 30 weeks gestation.

*The potential complications to the surviving twin in a monochorionic twin pregnancy are in the form of ischaemic brain damage, renal damage and increased mortality. The risk of coagulation disorder in the mother exists and requires monitoring. Management can be discussed under supportive, medical and surgical headings.*

The cause of death of one of the twins may be the hostile environment, which is a potential threat to the surviving twin.

### Prognosis                                                                    1 mark
Accurate timing of the fetal death in gestation is desirable.
Information pertaining to chorionicity is helpful in assessing the potential presence of placental anastomoses.

Communicating vessels are very uncommon in dichorionic gestations.              1 mark
The most significant problem is that the mortality and morbidity (46%) of the surviving twin is greatly increased in monochorionic twin pregnancy.

Up to 20–25% incidence of neurological damage, including cerebral palsy,        1 mark
porencephaly, hydrocephalus and cerebral infarction, has been noted in monochorionic twins.
Renal cortical necrosis may occur.

Disseminated intravascular coagulation (DIC) may affect as many as 25% of       1 mark
the mothers beyond 3 weeks of the demise.
Immediate and weekly assessment of coagulation studies of the mother is therefore necessary

### Supportive
Evaluation of fetal structural anomalies and frequent serial assessment of the  1 mark
status of the surviving twin using ultrasound, biophysical profile, cardiotocography is desirable.

The psychological status of the mother and her preferences should be taken      1 mark
into account before deciding the timing of delivery.

Neonatal cranial ultrasound is recommended after delivery, with magnetic        1 mark
resonance imaging (MRI) in the event of abnormality.

### Medical
Steroids are given to mother to prevent respiratory distress syndrome in the    1 mark
surviving fetus in case of premature delivery.

**Surgical**

To deliver the surviving twin, balancing the risks of prematurity versus risks of     1 mark
remaining *in utero* is necessary.
If preterm delivery is indicated for fetal reasons caesarean section is generally
the preferred route.

On balance, it is accepted that expectant management of the surviving twin     1 mark
should be adopted, especially when more time (>24 h) has elapsed since the
event.
This is because feto-fetal transfusion is an acute process following co-twin
death, as is the time course of ischaemic brain injury or death.

## Suggested reading

Enbom JA. Twin pregnancy with intrauterine death of one twin. *Am J Obstet Gynecol*
1985; 152: 424–9.

5. A primigravida attends at 38 weeks with confirmed spontaneous rupture of membranes and a singleton fetus in cephalic presentation. She is not in labour and has been well thus far. Critically evaluate your options of managing this patient.

*A good candidate will demonstrate the awareness of the two options, conservative management versus induction of labour, with their pros and cons. Manage according to the informed decision made by the woman.*

**Prognosis (background evidence for management options)**

Induction of labour (IOL) carries a lower risk of maternal and neonatal infection than expectant management. It may, however, increase use of pain relief and internal fetal heart monitoring. 1 mark

Many women feel more positive about IOL than expectant management. 1 mark

No statistical differences in outcome like caesarean section are observed with immediate or postponed induction, although there is a trend towards lesser interventions with expectant management. 1 mark

**Counselling**

Discussion of the options with the mother, and manage according to her wishes. 1 mark

**Management**
**Supportive**

Exclusion of infection: maternal temperature, pulse, white cell count, high vaginal swab, (C-reactive protein). 1 mark

Confirmation of fetal well-being: by cardiotocography; biophysical profile and Doppler when necessary. 1 mark

Conservative management if maternal and fetal well-being is confirmed is an option; most women (80–90%) will go into labour within 48 h after premature rupture of membranes. 1 mark

Twice-weekly review for maternal and fetal well-being can be done on outpatient basis until the patient goes into spontaneous labour. 1 mark

**Medical**

Induction of labour involves assessment of Bishop's score. 1 mark

There are few clinically significant differences between prostaglandin (PG) or oxytocin. 1 mark

Overall, PG is associated with less chance of epidural analgesia and a very slightly increased risk of chorioamnionitis and neonatal infection. There are no differences in neonatal outcome.

## Suggested reading

Tan BP, Hannah ME. Oxytocin for prelabour rupture of membranes at or near term [Cochrane Review], in The Cochrane Library, Issue 3, 2000. Oxford: Update software.

# PAPER 6: GYNAECOLOGY

1. What is the role of laparoscopy in hysterectomy? Discuss the advantages and disadvantages of laparoscopic hysterectomy.

2. Evaluate the return of fertility in a woman after discontinuation of contraception.

3. A primigravid woman presents at 9 weeks gestation with threatened miscarriage. An ultrasound scan reveals a live pregnancy in one horn of a bicornuate uterus with a single cervix. How would you counsel her?

4. A 25-year-old woman presents with a 2-year history of intermittent lower abdominal pain. She is sexually active. Enumerate the differential diagnosis and describe the appropriate diagnostic steps.

5. Justify the proposition for inclusion of human papillomavirus (HPV) testing in the cervical screening programme.

1. What is the role of laparoscopy in hysterectomy? Discuss the advantages and disadvantages of laparoscopic hysterectomy.

---

*A good candidate will discuss benefits and risks of using laparoscopy for hysterectomy. The role of laparoscopy is to convert an abdominal hysterectomy into a vaginal one that has lower morbidity. There is good evidence to show that the laparoscopic component should be kept to a minimum in a hysterectomy.*

### Role

The role of laparoscopy is to convert an abdominal hysterectomy into a vaginal hysterectomy.      1 mark

Vaginal hysterectomy is the hysterectomy that carries minimum morbidity and mortality amongst all the routes of hysterectomy.      1 mark

Laparoscopy at hysterectomy allows concurrent endometriosis and adhesions to be visualized and managed. This in turn allows the surgeon to perform a vaginal hysterectomy.      1 mark

In order to reduce the operative complications, the laparoscopic component should be kept to a minimum (i.e. defer bladder dissection and clamping the uterine arteries laparoscopically).      1 mark

### Advantages

Shorter hospital stay.      1 mark
Shorter recovery period and early return to work.

Reduced analgesic requirements.      1 mark
Better cosmetic scar than an abdominal hysterectomy.

Lower blood transfusion rates: allows strict haemostasis to be achieved.      1 mark

### Disadvantages

Costly equipment.      1 mark
Increased operation time.

Increased rate of ureteric injury.      1 mark
Higher rate of vesicovaginal fistula.
Incisional hernia.

Training and expertise, long learning curve.      1 mark
Other complications that can occur during a laparoscopy: anaesthetic, injury to other viscera.

## Suggested reading:

Meikle SF, Weston Nugent G.  Complications and recovery from laparoscopic assist-
    ed vaginal hysterectomy compared with abdominal and vaginal hysterectomy.
    *Obstet Gynecol* 1997; 89(2): 304–11.

2. Evaluate the return of fertility in a woman after discontinuation of contraception.

*A good candidate will discuss the delay, if any, in return of fertility in various methods of
contraception: natural, barrier, combined pills, minipills, Depo-Provera, implants, coil and
sterilization.*

### Combined oral contraceptive pill (COCP)

COCP is associated with ultimate return to fertility.                                1 mark
The post-pill delay in return of fertility is associated with the age of the
woman and the duration of use of the pill.

Post-pill amenorrhoea warrants investigation if it persists beyond 6 months       1 mark
after discontinuing COCP.
There is no increase in the rate of secondary amenorrhoea in previous pill
users.

There is an immediate return of fertility on discontinuing progesterone-only      1 mark
pills.

### Depo-Provera

The pregnancy rate in women after discontinuing Depo-Provera is normal            1 mark
(85% of women achieve conception within 24 months of discontinuation).
The delay to conception is about 9 months after the last injection, and the
delay does not increase with the duration of use.

### Implant

Most women resume normal ovulatory cycles during the first month after           1 mark
removal of Norplant.
There are no long-term effects on future fertility.

### Intrauterine contraceptive device (IUCD)

IUCD is associated with an increased incidence of pelvic inflammatory disease    1 mark
(PID) during the first 20 days after insertion. This may cause tubal infertility.

The decrease in the fertility rate is largely dependent on the lifestyle of the   1 mark
user. Infection beyond 20 days is mostly due to sexually transmitted infection.
The relative ectopic pregnancy (less than when not using any contraception
but more than when on COCP) may further reduce fertility.

### Levonorgestrel intrauterine system (LNG-IUS)

LNG-IUS does not appear to be associated with lowered fertility rates.           1 mark
This may be due to the lower incidence of PID and ectopic pregnancy
associated with it.

**Sterilization**

Tubal ligation is meant to be a permanent method of contraception, although          1 mark
it has a lifetime failure rate of 1 in 200 procedures.

The reversal of the procedure leads to a tubal patency rate of 70–80% and a
pregnancy rate of 40–60%.

Similarly, after reversal of vasectomy within 5 years, the fertility rate is about
40–60%.

**Natural methods**

Barrier and natural methods when discontinued are followed by the                      1 mark
immediate return of fertility.

3. A primigravid woman presents at 9 weeks gestation with threatened miscarriage. An ultrasound scan reveals a live pregnancy in one horn of a
bicornuate uterus with a single cervix. How would you counsel her?

*Remember this question is as much about miscarriage as about anomaly. Explanation of the
nature of problem, its association with urinary tract anomalies, range of possible outcomes
in pregnancy, need for increased surveillance and reassurance that majority of pregnancies
are uneventful.*

Explain the nature of the abnormality to the patient, with the aid of a diagram       1 mark

Reassure that most of the time, the outcome is favourable after a normal       1 mark
pregnancy and labour.

Explain a possible range of outcomes in early pregnancy, from a threatened       1 mark
miscarriage to uterine rupture, which is very rare, depending upon the details
of the severity of uterine malformation.

Explain the range of possible complications in late pregnancy: increased risk       3 marks
of preterm labour, intrauterine growth restriction, malpresentation, cord
prolapse, caesarean section, placental adherence.
(½ *mark for each complication mentioned*)

Explain the fact that there is no evidence that bedrest and hospitalization is       1 mark
beneficial for bleeding in early pregnancy.
If fetal heart is seen at the scan, the likelihood of continuation of pregnancy to
viability is good (90%).

Explain there is no need for increased antenatal surveillance.       1 mark

Explain the need for the exclusion of renal tract abnormalities with imaging       1 mark
techniques, such as ultrasound in pregnancy and intravenous urogram if
necessary after puerperium.

There is no need for surgical correction if the outcome in pregnancy is       1 mark
normal.
If there is recurrent mid-trimester losses, then operations such as Strassman's
or Tomkin's procedures can be attempted, but these are associated with
complications and do not guarantee successful pregnancy outcome.

## Suggested reading

Cooney MJ, Benson CB, Doubilet PM. Outcome of pregnancies in women with uterine duplication anomalies. *J Clin Ultrasound* 1998; 26(1): 3–6.

4. A 25-year-old woman presents with a 2-year history of intermittent lower abdominal pain. She is sexually active. Enumerate the differential diagnosis and describe the appropriate diagnostic steps.

*A good candidate will mention the gynaecological and non-gynaecological causes of chronic pelvic pain. The clinical approach should be in structured steps of history, examination, and investigations: non-invasive and invasive.*

The following diagnoses should be considered:

1. Endometriosis                                                                1 mark
2. Chronic pelvic inflammatory disease

3. Functional bowel disorders, e.g. irritable bowel syndrome, adhesions         1 mark
4. Pelvic congestion syndrome

5. Non-gynaecological causes, e.g. musculoskeletal, neurological,               1 mark
   urological and psychological causes

**History**

The patient is preferably seen in the pelvic pain clinic.                      1 mark
A good clinical history, including direct questions regarding gastrointestinal
symptoms. The onset, timing and quality of pain, as well as its relationship to
the menstrual cycle, is to be assessed.
History of sexual abuse in childhood, if suspected, is asked subtly and
sensitively.

Recognize that dyspareunia and cyclical symptoms may be a feature of non-       1 mark
gynaecological problems.
Psychological evaluation is recommended in occasional cases.

**Examination**

Thorough clinical examination: abdominal examination is necessary to rule       1 mark
out palpable pathology. Distended and tender caecum and sigmoid is
sometimes found in irritable bowel syndrome.

Pelvic examination is important, e.g. fixed retroversion, nodularity in the     1 mark
pouch of Douglas, cervical excitation, enlarged adnexa is significant.

**Investigations**

Nonsurgical relevant investigations, such as erythrocyte sedimentation rate     1 mark
(ESR), endocervical swabs for culture, urine microscopy, bowel studies
(Barium studies, colonoscopy) and intravenous urography.

Pelvic ultrasound scanning is of limited value, but it can be reassuring to the    1 mark
patient and sometimes may reveal pathology not noted on clinical examination.
Magnetic resonance imaging (MRI) is sometimes done for diagnosis of
rectovaginal septum endometriosis.

Laparoscopy carries risks and may lead to confounding diagnoses and    1 mark
erroneous treatment. It is the final step on the ladder of diagnostic
investigations.
In some women, the pain subsides after laparoscopy, the reason for which
cannot be explained.

## Suggested reading

Thomas EJ, Rock J. Pelvic pain, in *Benign Gynaecological Disease: Fast Facts*. Oxford: Health Press; 1997. pp. 34–8.

5. Justify the proposition for inclusion of human papillomavirus (HPV) testing in the cervical screening programme.

*A good candidate will discuss how HPV testing satisfies almost all the World Health Organization (WHO) screening criteria. Its utility in primary and secondary screening should be discussed.*

Cervical cancer is the second most common female genital tract cancer.          1 mark
Human papillomavirus (HPV) DNA is found in 95% of cervical carcinomas
and precursor lesions.

About 15–28% of HPV DNA-positive women with normal cytology develop          1 mark
cervical intraepithelial neoplasia (CIN) within 2 years compared with only
1–3% of HPV DNA-negative women.

The risk of progression is higher in the high-risk HPV types 16, 18 (and with          1 mark
probable carcinogenic strains of type 31, 33 and 35).
Viral load is a good predictor of persistent infection and hence higher degree
of CIN.

Combined cytology and HPV testing has a sensitivity of 96% and positive          1 mark
predictive value (PPV) of 64% for detecting CIN, and this may be improved by
subtype testing.
The positive predictive value of HPV for detection of CIN rises with age, while
that of cytology reduces.

Cost models estimate that HPV testing every decade could be cheaper and          1 mark
more sensitive than 3-yearly cervical smears.
It has been easily acceptable to women who undergo cervical screening.

The proposed value of testing for HPV DNA in primary screening is:

• As an adjunct to cytology in screening of women over the age of 35 years          1 mark
• Virus testing for the general population in developing countries without
  an organized screening programme.
• In women with mild dyskaryosis, referral to the colposcopy clinic          1 mark
  could be done if repeat HPV test after 6 months was found to be
  persistently positive.

The utility in secondary screening is:

• Resolution of low-grade cytology: approximately 75% of borderline          1 mark
  smears are in fact normal; the patient and clinician's anxiety can be

resolved through HPV DNA testing for the high-risk types
- Resolution of equivocal or low-grade histology (due to interobserver variation) can be resolved by the objective testing for HPV DNA

- Resolution of discrepancy between cytology and colposcopy 1 mark
- Test of cure: HPV testing following treatment can be used to ensure that both disease and HPV has been removed

## Suggested reading

Cuzick J, Sasieni P, Davies P *et al*. A systematic review of the role of human papillomavirus testing within a cervical screening programme. *Health Technol Assess* 1999; 3(14): 1–204.

# PAPER 7: OBSTETRICS

1. You see a 20-year-old pregnant woman in the booking clinic at 16 weeks of pregnancy. She admits to sniffing cocaine. Outline the plan of your management.

2. A woman who is 34 weeks pregnant and is diagnosed to have immune thrombocytopoenic purpura (ITP) is concerned about the effect of her condition on the fetus and the mode of delivery. What are the issues involved in care of this pregnancy?

3. A 28-year-old fit multipara was admitted to labour ward at 7-cm dilation at term with strong uterine contractions. After an hour of admission, she suddenly collapsed. There was no revealed bleeding and the uterus was soft. What are the likely diagnoses, and how should this woman be managed?

4. Debate the recent recommendation for offering HIV screening to all pregnant women.

4. Discuss the value of serial ultrasound scanning in pregnancy.

1. You see a 20-year-old pregnant woman in the booking clinic at 16 weeks of pregnancy. She admits to sniffing cocaine. Outline the plan of your management.

*A good candidate will draw a plan of management from the booking through to postnatal care, stressing on multidisciplinary care, screening for diseases associated with drugs, and addiction control.*

Multidisciplinary team approach providing obstetric, psychosocial and addiction management is necessary.

1 mark

### Antenatal care
An ultrasound scan is performed to confirm the gestation and then at mid-trimester to rule out fetal anomalies.
A vaginal swab is taken to screen for anaerobic vaginosis.

1 mark

Blood is taken to establish hepatitis B and hepatitis C status, and HIV test is offered.
The necessary precautions are taken if the woman is positive for HBsAg or HIV.
A genitourinary physician is involved in her care if positive for any of the above diseases.

1 mark

Drug history is taken and attainable targets are set. Methadone maintenance treatment is altered according to the drug diary maintained by the patient.

1 mark

Advising the patient regarding quitting use of cocaine is often counterproductive. Providing support as the targets are met is essential.

1 mark

Serial growth scans are arranged from 28 weeks every fortnight with assessment of liquor volume and umbilical artery Doppler studies from 34 weeks.

1 mark

A 'planning meeting' is held at around 32 weeks with the woman, her partner, the community drug team, the health visitor and social worker.
The needs of the mother and baby for the latter part of the pregnancy are discussed, as is the need for prenatal child protection.

1 mark

### Delivery
The requirement for opiates for pain relief in labour may be high due to tolerance.
A neonatologist should be present for the delivery.

1 mark

**Postnatal care**

After birth the baby is observed on the postnatal ward for signs of withdrawal.  1 mark

The mother and baby are discharged from the hospital after all the people  1 mark
involved are made aware of the same.
Contraception should be discussed before discharge.

## Suggested reading

Llewelyn R. Substance abuse in pregnancy: the team approach to antenatal care, *The Obstetrician and Gynaecologist.* 2000; 2(1): 11–15.

2. A woman who is 34 weeks pregnant and is diagnosed to have immune thrombocytopoenic purpura (ITP) is concerned about the effect of her condition on the fetus and the mode of delivery. What are the issues involved in care of this pregnancy?

*A good candidate should be able to discuss the pros and cons for vaginal delivery, instrumental delivery and lower segment caesarean section (LSCS). The monitoring of fetal platelet count post-delivery and administration of intravenous immunoglobulin if required should be discussed*

**Antenatal**

Before initiating any plan of treatment, advice from a physician with experience in dealing with this problem is sought.                    1 mark
Treatment is recommended in presence of platelet count <50 000/μl or bleeding complications.

Maternal serology and characteristics, including prior splenectomy, platelet     1 mark
count, and the presence of platelet-associated antibodies, all correlate poorly with neonatal thrombocytopenia.

Steroids and intravenous immunoglobulin (IVIG) do not reliably prevent           1 mark
fetal thrombocytopoenia or improve fetal outcome.
There is insufficient evidence to recommend maternal medical treatment for fetal indications.

There is increased risk (5%) of fetal intracranial haemorrhage when the count     1 mark
is less than 20 000/μl.

Cordocentesis carries a 1–2% risk of emergency caesarean delivery.               1 mark
The transfer of antiplatelet antibodies occurs at the end of pregnancy, so there is no place for serial fetal blood sampling.

There is a risk of inaccuracy and technical difficulty with fetal scalp blood     1 mark
sampling, so most obstetricians do not obtain fetal platelet counts.

**Delivery**

The mode of delivery in pregnancy complicated by ITP should be chosen            1 mark
based on obstetric considerations.

Epidural analgesia cannot be given when platelet count is below 50 000/μl.        1 mark
Fetal scalp monitoring, fetal scalp blood sampling and difficult instrumental delivery should be avoided in labour.

Caesarean section has not been shown to definitely reduce the risk of fetal       1 mark
intracranial haemorrhage.

**156**

If the maternal platelet count is less than 40 000/µl, then platelet transfusion is required if caesarean section is warranted (to avoid excessive bleeding).

**Postnatal**
Cord platelet count is determined immediately after delivery and neonatal          1 mark
platelet count is monitored over the next 3–4 days after delivery.
Intravenous immunoglobulin is given for neonates with bleeding or severe thrombocytopenia.

## Suggested reading

ACOG practice bulletin: thrombocytopenia in pregnancy. Number 6, September 1999. Clinical management guidelines for obstetrician–gynaecologists. *Int J Gynaecol Obstet* 1999; 67: 117–28.

3. A 28-year-old fit multipara was admitted to labour ward at 7-cm dilation at term with strong uterine contractions. After an hour of admission, she suddenly collapsed. There was no revealed bleeding and the uterus was soft. What are the likely diagnoses, and how should this woman be managed?

---

*A good candidate will discuss amniotic fluid embolism as the most likely diagnosis, followed by a list of other differential diagnoses. Investigations, monitoring and multidisciplinary care; supportive treatment should be promptly initiated. Prompt delivery of the patient is important.*

**Differential diagnoses**

Given the stage of labour, previous insignificant medical history, acute          1 mark
deterioration of the cardiorespiratory function and the lack of other
symptoms that may point to other differential diagnoses (chest pain, massive
bleeding), the most likely diagnosis is amniotic fluid embolism.

The other differential diagnoses include pulmonary embolism, air embolism,        1 mark
myocardial infarction, subarachnoid or cerebral haemorrhage, local
anaesthetic toxicity and septic shock.
(*1 mark for three or more differential diagnoses*)

**Investigations**

Full blood count, blood group and cross-match, clotting screen, urea and          2 marks
electrolytes, arterial blood gases, electrocardiogram, chest X-ray.
(*½ mark each for any four of the above*)

**Supportive treatment**

Invasive monitoring with central venous pressure line and preferably             1 mark
Swan–Ganz catheter.

Maintaining airway and oxygenation either via bag and mask or intubation          1 mark
and ventilation with 100% oxygen.

Cardiopulmonary resuscitation with the possible use of inotropes.                 1 mark
Maintaining the cardiac output with colloids and blood.

**Multidisciplinary care**

Early involvement of senior obstetrical, anaesthetic and haematological staff      1 mark
should be sought.
Patient should be transferred to ITU for care in collaboration with the
intensivists after delivery.

**Medical treatment**

If coagulopathy develops, it needs to be corrected with whole blood, fresh         1 mark
frozen plasma, platelets and cryoprecipitate after consultation with the
haematologist.
Use of heparin is controversial.

**Surgical treatment**

Immediate delivery (by caesarean section if necessary) after stabilizing the        1 mark
woman is necessary.

## Suggested reading

Clark SL, Hankins GD, Dudley DA *et al.* Amniotic fluid embolism: analysis of the
national registry. *Am J Obstet Gynecol* 1995; 172: 1158–69.

4. Debate the recent recommendation for offering HIV screening to all pregnant women.

*A good candidate will discuss the benefits of HIV screening in pregnancy. Do not forget to mention the drawbacks and how they can be minimized.*

Screening allows appropriate management options in screen-positive individuals as early HIV detection can have benefits.

### Medical
One of the main reasons for determining HIV status in pregnancy is to reduce vertical transmission.                                                                                    1 mark
The administration of zidovudine and nevirapine antenatally and during delivery and to the newborn infant reduces this rate by two-thirds in women who are HIV positive.

Breastfeeding doubles the rate of vertical transmission. In the UK, 77% of women diagnosed after delivery breastfeed compared with 4% of those diagnosed before delivery.                                                                               1 mark
This demonstrates that knowing the HIV status before delivery is helpful in avoiding breastfeeding and thereby in reducing the rate of transmission.

A newborn infant who is HIV positive should receive anti-retroviral treatment and prophylactic antibiotics against pneumocystis pneumonia to improve prognosis.                                                                                    1 mark

The health risk to healthcare professionals is reduced if appropriate precautions are taken while caring for HIV-positive individuals.                              1 mark

### Surgical
Caesarean section may reduce the vertical transmission rate.                        1 mark

Avoidance of invasive procedures during delivery (e.g. fetal scalp electrode, fetal scalp blood sampling) may reduce the risk of vertical transmission.           1 mark

About 20% of women who are diagnosed HIV positive during pregnancy choose to terminate the pregnancy.                                                         1 mark

### Supportive
As well as deciding about current pregnancy, the woman can make decisions regarding her future fertility and can take steps to reduce the risk of transmission of HIV to her partner.                                                     1 mark

The emotional trauma can be devastating, but can be helped tremendously by proper counselling. There are other adverse social and financial                     1 mark implications, which can be minimized by appropriate counselling and social awareness.

These considerations favour recommending testing for HIV to every woman          1 mark
in pregnancy. There is no discrimination against high-risk groups, and acceptance by women is higher. Mandatory testing may deter women from attending for antenatal care and is counterproductive, hence opt-in testing is the recommendable alternative.

## Suggested reading

Brocklehurst, P. Interventions aimed at decreasing the risk of mother-to-child transmission of HIV infection [systematic review], In The Cochrane Library, Issue 3, 2000. Oxford: Update software.

Merccy D, Nicoll A. We should routinely offer HIV screening in pregnancy. *Br J Obstet Gynaecol* 1998; 105: 249–51.

5. Discuss the value of serial ultrasound scanning in pregnancy.

*A good candidate will discuss the use of serial ultrasound scanning during pregnancy to monitor threatened miscarriage viability and resolution of early pregnancy bleeding; structural defects and multiple pregnancies (mid- and late-trimester); abnormalities of amniotic fluid and fetal growth (late pregnancy).*

Serial ultrasound scanning (USS) is not necessary for successful completion of a low-risk pregnancy. — 1 mark

Threatened miscarriage with potential non-viable pregnancy: scan repeated in 1–2 weeks allows growth to be detected by high-frequency transvaginal scan. Serial USS performed at this time is used to document the normal progression of intrauterine pregnancy or the resolution of intrauterine bleeding. — 1 mark

Follow-up of confirmed fetal abnormalities: fetal congenital heart disease and hydronephrosis and hydrocephalus where the degree of obstruction may worsen with advancing gestational age. — 1 mark

Follow-up examination is often requested if insufficient imaging of the fetus is obtained at the initial evaluation.
They have a low yield, however, in detecting fetal structural abnormalities in the organ system, that was imaged inadequately during the initial study. — 1 mark

In cases with increased risk of fetal demise (high-risk pregnancies, such as gestational diabetes, intrahepatic cholestasis of pregnancy, pre-eclampsia), biophysical profile (BPP) is performed up to two to three times a week to evaluate a fetus at increased risk of stillbirth. — 1 mark

Abnormalities of fetal growth can be picked up in patients who are at risk of fetal growth restriction, fetal macrosomia by serial scans. — 1 mark

Abnormalities of fetal amniotic fluid: in case of oligohydramnios, amniotic fluid index, fetal growth and Dopplers are serially monitored and the endpoint is usually induction of labour for the fear of fetal demise. — 1 mark

In polyhydramnios, the serial ultrasound examinations are used to determine the risk of preterm labour and the need for medical treatment. — 1 mark

Growth of multiple gestations can be properly monitored with USS done every 4 weeks from 24 weeks. — 1 mark
Monochorionic twin pregnancy requires more intensive monitoring than dichorionic twin pregnancy. — 1 mark

## Suggsted reading

http://www.atlanta-mfm.com/clindisc/fu_ultra.html.

# PAPER 7: GYNAECOLOGY

1. Taking the natural history into consideration, justify the management options for a patient with vulval intraepithelial neoplasia (VIN).

2. A 23-year-old girl comes to the clinic complaining of worsening hirsutism, which interferes with her personal and social life. How would you manage her case?

3. Discuss the use of mifepristone in medical termination of pregnancy, and mention other possible indications for this drug in obstetrics and gynaecology.

4. Discuss the role of laparoscopy in different disorders presenting with acute pelvic pain of gynaecological origin in a woman of reproductive age group in whom pregnancy is excluded.

5. How will you counsel a couple who have decided to undergo *in vitro* fertilization (IVF) regarding the risks of the treatment?

1. Taking the natural history into consideration, justify the management options for a patient with vulval intraepithelial neoplasia (VIN).

*There is a higher risk of invasion in postmenopausal, immunosuppressed women with uni-focal lesions. Colposcopy, biopsy and histopathology should be done to exclude malignancy. Conservative management with long-term follow-up is appropriate in young women with multifocal disease. 5- fluorouracil and interferon are not of substantial value. Wide local excision is recommended if the risk of invasion is high. Few patients require more radical surgery.*

**Natural history**

VIN may be multifocal or unifocal.                                      1 mark
The risk of invasive disease is small after VIN, and majority occurs in women who are postmenopausal and have unifocal lesions.

Those women who have immunosuppression, i.e. renal transplants, lupus          1 mark
erythematosus, Fanconi's anaemia and those who have multifocal lower genital tract neoplasia are at higher risk of vulval carcinoma and should be treated.

**Investigations**

Examination of lower genital tract to rule out other premalignant or            1 mark
malignant disease is carried out.
Colposcopy, biopsy and histopathology should be done to exclude malignancy.

Excisional biopsy is recommended in hyperkeratotic, pigmented, elevated,        1 mark
irregular lesions, and those with abnormal vascular pattern or progressive severity.

**Treatment**
**Supportive**

Regression of VIN is seen when the diagnosis is made in young and/or           1 mark
pregnant woman with multifocal disease.
In such cases, conservative management is permissible in anticipation of regression.

Long-term follow-up is necessary, keeping in mind the natural history of the    1 mark
disease.
Rebiopsy of suspicious areas is essential to detect invasive disease in those who relapse.

**Medical**

Drug treatment includes topical 5-fluorouracil, alfa interferon and            1 mark
dinitrochlorobenzene. None of these have proven to be of substantial benefit, and all are associated with severe reactions.

**Surgical**

In $CO_2$ laser vaporization, tissue is destroyed up to the upper reticular dermis.   1 mark
Apart from the cost-effectiveness, nonavailability of tissue for histopathology
and high rate of recurrence (70%) have put this option out of favour.

When the risk of invasion is high, wide local excision with 1-cm margin of   1 mark
normal tissue is required. Histopathology of the resected margins is advisable.

In a few patients, more radical surgery may be required with some requiring   1 mark
skin grafting; this is better managed in units experienced in the management
of this condition.
Psychosexual counselling and support may be desirable in some patients who require
repeated surgery.

## Suggested reading

Acheson N, Ganesan R, Chan KK. Premalignant vulval disorders. *Curr Obstet
Gynaecol* 2000; 10: 12–17.

2. A 23-year-old girl comes to the clinic complaining of worsening hirsutism, which interferes with her personal and social life. How would you manage her case?

*A good candidate will structure the answer as per the usual clinical approach of history, examination, investigations and treatment – supportive, medical and surgical.*

**History and examination**                                    1 mark
Timing of onset, breast changes, distribution of hirsutism, weight gain, menstrual changes etc.

**Laboratory investigations**
Total serum testosterone concentration (> 6 nmol/l is highly suggestive of       1 mark
neoplastic cause), androstenedione, dehydroepiandrosterone.
LH, FSH, prolactin, thyroid function tests if associated menstrual disturbances.

Pelvic ultrasonography to look for ovarian morphology typical of polycystic       1 mark
ovaries

**Supportive treatment**
Weight loss.                                                    1 mark

Cosmetic approaches: shaving, depilation, bleaching, electrolysis therapy.       1 mark

**Psychological management**
It is necessary to counsel her regarding long treatment time to achieve          1 mark
response, side-effect profile, contraception whilst on anti-androgen medication
and non-permanent nature of the therapy.

**Pharmacological treatment**
Combined oral contraceptives: less androgenic, such as Cilest or one             2 marks
containing cyproterone acetate (Dianette); most suitable if contraception is
also desired.

Cyproterone acetate, spironolactone.                                            1 mark
Other anti-androgens that can be used but have serious side-effect profiles are
flutamide and ketoconazole.

**Surgical treatment**
This is dependent on diagnosis. Hypophysectomy for Cushing's syndrome due        1 mark
to hyperplasia, removal of adrenal or ovarian tumours or corticosteroids for
virilizing adrenal hyperplasia.
There is no role for surgery in idiopathic hirsutism.

## Suggested reading

Conn J, Jacobs HS. Managing hirsutism in gynaecological practice. *Br J Obstet Gynaecol* 1998; 105: 687–96.

3. Discuss the use of mifepristone in medical termination of pregnancy, and mention other possible indications for this drug in obstetrics and gynaecology.

---

*Discuss the indications, contraindications and procedure of first-trimester medical termina-tion along with follow-up. The other uses include mid-trimester and third-trimester termi-nation, cervical priming, contraception, and in gynaecological disorders such as fibroids, endometriosis, as adjunct in cancer treatment, and in research.*

Mifepristone (RU 486) can be used up to nine completed weeks of pregnancy    1 mark
(63 days of amenorrhoea), and when used in conjunction with prostaglandin
is associated with up to 95–97% success rates.

It is given in the form of a single oral dose of 600 mg or 200 mg (unlicensed    1 mark
dose but similar efficacy) followed 36–48 h later by gemeprost (Cervagem)
1 mg vaginally. The patient is observed for 6 h.

Contraindications to RU 486: smokers over 35 years, steroids, porphyria,    1 mark
adrenal failure, bleeding disorders.

The possible side effects are painful cramps requiring analgesia, prolonged    1 mark
bleeding, incomplete termination requiring suction and curettage.

Follow-up is arranged 8–14 days later to exclude on-going pregnancy and to    1 mark
confirm completeness of the procedure.

For mid-trimester abortion, mifepristone 600 mg orally followed 36–48 h later    1 mark
by gemeprost 1 mg vaginally repeated every 3 h to a maximum of five
pessaries in 24h.

## Other potential uses
There are a few studies indicating that it could be useful in termination of    1 mark
pregnancy (TOP) up to 83 days of amenorrhoea.
TOP in third trimester and induction of labour.

## Contraception
Treatment after a single act of unprotected intercourse (postcoital    1 mark
contraception), and once-a-month treatment immediately after ovulation, has
shown high contraceptive efficacy. It is not yet licensed for this use.

**Leiomyoma**: potential to treat symptomatic uterine fibroids.    1 mark
**Ectopic pregnancy**: there is some evidence that the combination of
mifepristone and methotrexate decreases the risk of failure in medical
treatment of ectopic pregnancy.

**Endometriosis**: in extensive endometriosis, mifepristone is indicated for    1 mark
intractable pain, although its effect on the lesions will be minimal.
**Research**: RU 486 is a powerful tool to study the molecular action of
progesterone, and in the future may be used as an oestrogen-free contraceptive.
**Adjuvant therapy in cancer**: e.g. management of unresectable and metastatic
breast cancer.
(*1 mark for mentioning any two of the above*)

## Suggested reading

The care of woman requesting induced abortion. *Evidence Based Guideline No. 7*,
    RCOG. Clinical Effectiveness Support Unit. London: RCOG Press; 2000.

Koide SS. Mifepristone: auxillary therapeutic use in cancer and related disorders. *J
    Reprod Med*. 1998; 43(7): 551–60.

4. Discuss the role of laparoscopy in different disorders presenting with acute pelvic pain of gynaecological origin in a woman of reproductive age group in whom pregnancy is excluded.

*A good candidate will demonstrate the knowledge of use of laparoscopy in diagnosis and treatment of pelvic inflammatory disease (PID), tubo-ovarian abscess, adnexal torsion. No marks will be allotted for ectopic pregnancy.*

Thorough history and examination is essential to rule out non-gynaecological causes and make a provisional diagnosis in case of gynaecological pain. Laparoscopy allows rapid diagnosis. This leads to early or concurrent treatment options to prevent sequel from the various problems.
1 mark

### Pelvic inflammatory disease (PID)
Early diagnosis and prompt treatment are necessary to prevent the chronic sequel, such as infertility, ectopic pregnancy and chronic pelvic pain.
1 mark

Laparoscopy currently represents the gold standard for the diagnosis of PID. It should be used when the diagnosis is uncertain and for patients who have not responded to antibiotics within 48–72 h.
1 mark

Any fluid should be aspirated, and biopsy samples should be obtained from infected or inflammed tissues for culture.
The surgical steps in pelvic abscess include adhesiolysis, aspiration of the abscess cavity, excision of necrotic tissue, and thorough irrigation of the peritoneal cavity before completion of the procedure.
1 mark

### Tubo-ovarian abscess
Women with acute or subacute onset of lower abdominal pain and a pelvic mass that is either palpable or detected at ultrasound require early laparoscopy for confirmation of the diagnosis and institution of treatment.
1 mark

Laparoscopic surgery (drainage of abscess/removal of diseased organs) combined with adequate broad-spectrum antibiotic therapy is proven successful in the treatment of 95% of cases.
1 mark

### Adnexal torsion
The most common causes are benign ovarian tumours and cysts; malignant ones are rare. Torsion of a normal tube or tubal stump as after sterilization is rare. The diagnosis can be made only at laparoscopy or laparotomy.
1 mark

Conservative approach is best when tissues are viable, and should be carried out promptly to preserve the adnexa, the principle being to untwist the structure and treat the underlying cause, e.g. remove the cyst.
1 mark

Complete removal of the tube or ovary or both is necessary in the presence of     1 mark
irreversible damage.

**Contraindications**
Patients who are haemodynamically unstable, with cardiorespiratory disorders,     1 mark
and relatively contraindicated in patient with multiple scars on the abdomen.

## Suggested reading

Knudsen UB, Agaard J. Acute pelvic pain, in J Studd (ed.) *Progress in Obstetrics and Gynaecology* 13. London: Churchill Livingstone; 1999. pp. 311–23.

Porpora MG, Gomel V. The role of laparoscopy in the management of pelvic pain in women of reproductive age. *Fertility and Sterility* 1997; 68(5): 765–79.

5. How will you counsel a couple who have decided to undergo *in vitro* fertilization (IVF) regarding the risks of the treatment?

*A good candidate will discuss the following risks and preventive strategies where possible: ovarian hyperstimulation, cycle cancellation, potential of damaging the viscera and introducing pelvic infection by oocyte retrieval, risk of congenital anomalies with intracytoplasmic sperm injection (ICSI), multiple pregnancy and its complications, ectopic pregnancy and laboratory problems as well as financial, emotional and time burdens.*

Ovarian hyperstimulation: excess stimulation of ovaries can be a deliberate consequence of the treatment in order to maximize the yield of eggs. Monitoring aims to prevent this, but the patient should be aware of the symptoms and let the medical staff know if and when they arise.                    1 mark

The majority of cases are mild and settle in a few days. Occasionally, the problem may be a severe one requiring hospitalization and further treatment.        1 mark

Occasionally, the stimulation cycle can be abandoned due to poor stimulation or excessive stimulation.                                                       1 mark
The treatment can cause financial, emotional and time burdens.
The risk of adverse reactions to the anaesthetic or sedation is small.

Risk of damage to bowel, bladder and blood vessels during egg collection is small.                                                                          1 mark
If this occurs, an immediate abdominal operation is required to correct the problem.

Risk of pelvic infection due to egg collection is small. This is minimized by screening with genital swabs and prophylactic antibiotics before oocyte retrieval.                                                                       1 mark
The treatment does not increase the risk of miscarriage.

Intracytoplasmic sperm injection (ICSI) treatment carries a slightly increased chance of congenital abnormality, especially of Y chromosome in a male baby.   1 mark

Occasionally, there can be laboratory problems, such as failure of fertilization and poor quality of embryos.                                                 1 mark
Although embryo transfer is a relatively simple procedure, rarely one or more of the embryos may be lost in the transfer process.

The risk of ectopic pregnancy in IVF is higher than in the background population (3% v. 0.5%).                                                         1 mark
Heterotopic pregnancy can occur in 1 in 200 cases undergoing IVF.

The incidence of multiple pregnancy is much higher in IVF treatment. The complications of multiple pregnancy are higher rate of miscarriage, congenital anomalies, prematurity, maternal medical and obstetric complications. It can also present social and financial burdens on the family.
(*allot ½ mark each for any four of the above complications*)

2 marks

The risk can be reduced to some extent by restricting the number of embryos transferred to two.

# PAPER 8: OBSTETRICS

1. What processes will you ensure are in place for good risk management in your delivery suite?

2. How would you ensure that the caesarean section rate in labour in your hospital is kept to a minimum, consistent with good practice?

3. A 28-year-old primigravida attends the booking clinic at 11 weeks gestation. She weighs 127 kg and her body mass index is 38. She has no other risk factors of note. How does this affect her care in pregnancy, labour and puerperium?

4. A 23-year-old primigravida is diagnosed to have idiopathic polyhydramnios at 27 weeks gestation. Appraise the treatment available for this condition.

5. A 25-year-old primiparous patient requires caesarean section. On entry into the abdomen, a 4-cm hole is made in the bladder. Discuss the management and the issues you discuss with the patient.

1.  What processes will you ensure are in place for good risk management in your delivery suite?

*A good candidate will discuss risk identification, risk analysis, risk control and funding, which are the essential aspects of good risk management in the delivery suite.*

### Purpose
The purpose of risk management is to ensure that harm to patients, relatives and staff is avoided at the workplace. When mishaps occur, the potential for damage is to be minimized.                                        1 mark

### Risk identification
Reporting 'near-misses' by means of incident forms, the lessons learnt are disseminated to avoid recurrence.                                          1 mark

### Risk analysis
An expert committee can review a selected percentage of the reported incidents.                                                               1 mark
Clinical committees (labour ward forum, obstetric risk management group) comprising an obstetrician, anaesthetist, neonatologist, midwife representative, trainees representative, risk manager and consumer representative is set up to ensure good practice.

### Risk control
The labour ward protocols, clinical care pathways and guidelines should be updated regularly. Junior doctors need to be introduced to these at induction.    1 mark

There must be regular teaching, training and fire drills for the junior staff and midwives.                                                              1 mark

Adequate staffing levels (i.e. 40-h labour ward consultant cover, 1.15 midwives per woman in labour, and junior staffing) should be ensured.                 1 mark

Accurate documentation in notes is to be encouraged. All entries should be dated, signed and printed.                                              1 mark
Storing all old labour ward protocols, old timetables and rotas is essential. This should be the responsibility of a named individual.

Good communication is the best strategy to prevent complaints. Clear explanation to the patient and her partner for the intervention and follow-up visit the next day is good practice.                                            1 mark

Efficient complaints procedure can avoid a lot of litigation.                   1 mark

Regular clinical audits in order to monitor and improve standards are necessary in accordance with clinical governance.                            1 mark

## Suggested reading

Irvine LM. Practical risk management advice on the labour ward, in J Studd (ed.) *Progress in Obstetrics and Gynaecology*, 12. London: Churchill Livingstone; p. 59–65.

RCOG. Clinical risk management for obstetricians and gynaecologists. *Clinical Governance Advice No. 2*. London: RCOG Press; 2000.

2. How would you ensure that the caesarean section rate in labour in your hospital is kept to a minimum, consistent with good practice?

*A good candidate should enumerate the antepartum and intrapartum measures that can help to reduce unnecessary caesarean sections. Auditing the practice against set guidelines helps to improve practice.*

Caesarean section is a major procedure associated with maternal morbidity and mortality. Overintervention can be risky, and appropriate measures to reduce this attitude are in order.

### Antepartum
Labour ward guidelines and protocols based on evidence should be agreed upon and followed to ensure optimum outcome for the mother and her fetus (e.g. offering external cephalic version for singleton breech presentation without any contraindication for the procedure). 1 mark

Multidisciplinary education of all staff involved in the care of a parturient. 1 mark

One-to-one midwifery support with antenatal preparation. 1 mark

### Intrapartum
Correct diagnosis of labour (active phase) helps reduce caesarean sections in latent phases, as for failure to progress or failed induction. 1 mark

Routine amniotomy should not be performed because it does not improve outcome and is associated with cardiotocograph (CTG) artefacts.
Active management of labour does not reduce the caesarean section rates. 1 mark

Continuous fetal monitoring should be restricted to high-risk pregnancies. 1 mark

Fetal distress on CTG should be confirmed by fetal scalp blood sampling. 1 mark

Every effort should be made to correct uterine hypotonia before resorting to caesarean section for dystocia. 1 mark

The oxytocin infusion increment regimen should be every 30 min to avoid risks of hyperstimulation. 1 mark

### Postpartum
Audit the practice against set standards to highlight gaps and address them. 1 mark

## Suggested reading

Enkin M, Keirse MJNC, Renfrew M, Neilson J. Prolonged labour, in *Guide to Effective Care in Pregnancy and Childbirth*, 2nd edn. Oxford: Oxford University Press; 1998. pp. 262–8.

3. A 28-year-old primigravida attends the booking clinic at 11 weeks gestation. She weighs 127 kg and her body mass index is 38. She has no other risk factors of note. How does this affect her care in pregnancy, labour and puerperium?

*A good candidate should recognize the risks associated with obesity in pregnancy and suggest preventive measures: increased predisposition to difficulty in determining fetal heart and fetal growth clinically, gestational diabetes, and pre-eclampsia. Intrapartum risks include those of anaesthesia and shoulder dystocia. Postpartum risks are those of deep vein thrombosis, delayed wound healing and haematoma.*

**Antenatal**

Clinical diagnosis of pregnancy can sometimes be difficult. *1 mark*
As the pregnancy proceeds, it may be equally difficult to evaluate the size of the fetus, determine the presenting fetal part, detect fetal heart, or recognize the presence or absence of hydramnios.

Maternal blood pressure is difficult to determine when the maternal upper *1 mark*
arm is fat.
Large cuffs should be used for these women to avoid falsely high or low readings.

Dietary restriction of women for excessive weight gain can impair fetal growth *1 mark*
and result in height and weight deficit in the child, hence it is not advisable.
If there is suspicion of growth restriction, serial ultrasound should be arranged.

Latent diabetes is common in obese women of increasing age. *1 mark*
Arrange for glucose tolerance test at 26 weeks to uncover latent diabetes.

**Intrapartum**

It can be mechanically difficult to site an infusion in a fat limb and to site an *1 mark*
epidural cannula.
If there are any problems anticipated, siting a cannula in advance is desirable.

If caesarean section is required, both surgery and anaesthesia is hazardous in *1 mark*
such women. Delayed healing due to sweating or haematoma formation is more common in obese women.

The involvement of the most senior obstetrician and anaesthetist on site is *1 mark*
desirable.
Adequate asepsis and haemostasis, prophylactic antibiotics and hygiene are the usual precautions to prevent infection.

Low Apgar score and macrosomia are more frequent in women who are *1 mark*
overweight.

Regular drills and protocols help the labour ward to be prepared for shoulder dystocia in such a patient.

**Postpartum**
Obesity is a risk factor for deep vein thrombosis.                              1 mark
Early ambulation post-delivery should be encouraged.
Thromboembolic deterrent stockings and heparin prophylaxis if operative delivery required.

Tight control of weight before next pregnancy is advised. Combined oral          1 mark
contraceptives are a relative contraindication.

## Suggested reading

Galtier-Dereure F, Boegner C, Bringer J. Obesity and pregnancy: complications and cost (review). *Am J Clin Nutr* 2000 71(5 suppl): 1292–8.

4. A 23-year-old primigravida is diagnosed to have idiopathic polyhydramnios at 27 weeks gestation. Appraise the treatment available for this condition.

*A good candidate will know that the aim of treatment is to alleviate maternal discomfort and reduce the risk of preterm labour. Mild polyhydramnios does not need treatment, only monitoring. Use of indomethacin is the medical option. A course of corticosteroids is administered in case of threatened preterm labour. Serial amnioreduction is done for severe idiopathic polyhydramnios. Elective induction of labour or caesarean section are the options for delivery. Active management of third stage helps to reduce the risk of postpartum haemorrhage.*

### Antepartum
The aim of treatment is to relieve maternal discomfort and reduce the risk of preterm labour by reduction of the increased intrauterine pressure.          1 mark

### Supportive
Mild asymptomatic polyhydramnios (defined as a vertical amniotic fluid          1 mark
pocket greater than 8 cm but less than 12 cm) does not need treatment.
Dietary salt restriction has no benefit, and diuretics are potentially harmful.
(*allot ½ mark each for these points*)

Fetal growth needs to be monitored by serial ultrasound scans (USS).          1 mark
The combination of small for gestational age and hydramnios is a risk factor
for intrapartum complications and perinatal mortality, even in the absence of
congenital malformations.

### Medical
One option for treatment is the use of prostaglandin synthetase inhibitors.          1 mark
Indomethacin acts by decreasing fetal urinary output or by increasing the
reabsorption of fluid via the lungs.

The treatment should be suspended at 32 weeks gestation to avoid neonatal          1 mark
haemodynamic complications, such as premature closure of ductus arteriosus.
Periodic surveillance during treatment to search for signs of ductal
constriction, such as tricuspid regurgitation, is warranted.

A course of corticosteroids should be administered to the mother if delivery is          1 mark
anticipated before 36 weeks.

### Surgical
Serial amniotic fluid decompression (amnioreduction) is the treatment of          1 mark
choice for severe polyhydramnios (defined as a vertical pocket greater than
16 cm).

The disadvantages include the risk of preterm premature rupture of          1 mark
membranes, chorioamnionitis, abruptio placentae and onset of preterm
labour. It needs to be done under USS guidance every time.

### Delivery
Induction of labour may be required after 36 weeks. It carries the risk of cord          1 mark
prolapse and abruption.
Lower segment caesarean section (LSCS) is safer if done as an elective
procedure in severe polyhydramnios.

### Postpartum
Active management of third stage of labour reduces the risk of postpartum          1 mark
haemorrhage.

## Suggested reading

Cardwell M. Polyhydramnios: a review. *Obstet Gynecol Surv* 1987; 42(10): 612–17.

5. A 25-year-old primiparous patient requires caesarean section. On entry into the abdomen, a 4-cm hole is made in the bladder. Discuss the management and the issues you discuss with the patient.

*A good candidate will describe the repair technique, precautions and postoperative care and counselling involved with this complication.*

### Intraoperative management
The first step is to complete the delivery.                                    1 mark
After the uterus is sutured, extent of injury is delineated.

Ureteric catheterization is done if the tear is close to the ureters to ensure that    1 mark
they are safe and are not included in the subsequent suturing.

There is no clear evidence of the advantage of one repair technique over              1 mark
another (locked v. unlocked, single v. double layer, interrupted v. continuous
sutures).

Suture material of choice currently is vicryl 2/0.                               1 mark

Suprapubic catheterization is preferred over urethral catheter, and is kept *in*       1 mark
*situ* for 5–10 days.

Extraperitonization of the repaired site with drainage.                          1 mark

If the tear appears difficult to repair, or it is near the ureteric orifice,            1 mark
involvement of urologist is desirable.

### Postoperative care
Monitor urine output for first 24–48 h.                                         1 mark

### Counselling
The nature and the cause of the problem are explained to the patient, along           1 mark
with the importance of drainage.
Explain the slightly higher risk of urinary tract infection because of prolonged
catheterization, but no long-term residual effect.

As far as future deliveries are concerned, trial of vaginal delivery can be           1 mark
planned if there is no contraindication for the same.
Caution needs to be maintained in all future surgeries.

# PAPER 8: GYNAECOLOGY

1. Describe the measures that can be taken to decrease perioperative morbidity and mortality in gynaecological surgery.

2. Discuss your management of a 21-year-old woman who presents with secondary amenorrhoea and serum prolactin of 2800 IU/l.

3. A 50-year-old woman who has been diagnosed to have detrusor instability in your urodynamics clinic and is otherwise fit is seeking treatment, as this condition affects her quality of life to a great extent. How will you advise her regarding available treatment options?

4. A 50-year-old woman undergoes hysterectomy with bilateral oophorectomy for stage Ia poorly differentiated endometrial cancer. She wishes to commence hormone replacement therapy (HRT). How will you counsel her regarding the pros and cons of HRT?

5. Debate the proposition of introducing selective chlamydia screening in the UK.

1. Describe the measures that can be taken to decrease perioperative morbidity and mortality in gynaecological surgery.

*A good candidate will include the following points: ensuring correct indication, anaesthetic fitness, prevention of deep vein thrombosis (DVT) and infection, training and supervision of the staff, designated theatres and teams, guidelines, audits and Confidential Enquiry into Peri-Operative Deaths (CEPOD).*

**Preoperative**

Make sure that the operation is genuinely indicated (is the operation necessary?).                                                                1 mark

Ensure that the patient is fit for surgery by controlling the medical problems.   1 mark

Correct choice of anaesthesia is important to reduce morbidity, so it is desirable to ensure that the patient has a preoperative anaesthetic review.    1 mark

**Intraoperative**

Reduction in the rate of infection can be achieved by routine use of antibiotic prophylaxis for major procedures.                              1 mark

Having trained staff (medical and nursing) with adequate supervision at all levels helps to reduce mishaps.                                      1 mark

Morbidity can also be reduced by correct and timely decisions, and early involvement of senior staff, i.e. consultant.                          1 mark

Having designated theatre time, surgeon and team (for procedures such as evacuation of retained products of conception, ectopic pregnancy in a haemodynamically stable patient) helps reduce the number of procedures done at night and the morbidity associated with emergency surgery.   1 mark

**Postoperative**

Prevention of deep vein thrombosis (DVT) and pulmonary embolism by early mobilization, adequate hydration, thromboembolic deterrent stockings and heparin is essential.                                              1 mark

Setting up guidelines helps in appropriate management of surgical cases. Regular audit spirals for identifying high-risk areas and taking appropriate steps helps to improve practice.                                   1 mark

Confidential enquiry into perioperative deaths are audits done at a national level that help set national standards and provide uniformly excellent service.   1 mark

## Suggested reading

CEPOD: **http://www.ncepod.org.uk/dhome.htm**.

2. Discuss your management of a 21-year-old woman who presents with secondary amenorrhoea and serum prolactin of 2800 IU/l.

*A good candidate should be able to diagnose and manage the problem in the structured format of history, examination, investigations and treatment – supportive, medical and surgical.*

### History
Including menstrual history, drug history (phenothiazines), lactation and stress.                                                                                1 mark

History of medical disorders such as hypothyroidism and renal or hepatic dysfunction is sought.                                                                    1 mark
Association with polycystic ovaries is suggested by other symptoms such as hirsutism and infertility.

### Examination
To look for thyroid enlargement, galactorrhoea and secondary sexual characteristics.                                                                           1 mark

### Investigations
Pregnancy test or ultrasound scan (USS) to exclude pregnancy.                       1 mark

Pituitary imaging: computer-assisted tomography (CT) scan/magnetic resonance imaging (MRI)/X-ray skull):                                                       1 mark

- Microadenoma – pituitary neoplasm 5–10 mm in size
- Macroadenoma – over 10 mm in size
- Hyperprolactinaemia – <5 mm in size

### Treatment
### Supportive
In case of macroprolactinomas and suprasellar extension repeat pituitary imaging is advisable after a few months of medical treatment.                          1 mark
Treatment is advisable to reduce the risk of osteoporosis, if she wishes fertility, or if the prolactinoma is producing visual and other symptoms.

If patient is seeking pregnancy, the advice is to discontinue barrier contraception when tumour shrinkage is demonstrated on the follow-up scan and bromocriptine is discontinued as soon as pregnancy is confirmed (the risk of tumour expansion in pregnancy is less than 5%).                                    1 mark

### Medical
Bromocriptine normalizes prolactin in more than 90% of patients and shrinks 80% of macroprolactinomas.                                                          1 mark

Cabergoline is the drug of choice. It has twice-weekly dosage and fewer side- 1 mark
effects than bromocriptine, although it is a costlier drug.

**Surgical**
Macroadenoma with a serum prolactin <3000 IU/l needs surgical removal as it 1 mark
is likely to be nonfunctional.

## Suggested reading

Soule SG, Jacobs HS. Advances in the management of prolactinomas. *PACE Review No. 96/07*. London: RCOG Press; 1996.

3. A 50-year-old woman who has been diagnosed to have detrusor instability in your urodynamics clinic and is otherwise fit is seeking treatment, as
   this condition affects her quality of life to a great extent. How will you
   advise her regarding available treatment options?

*A good candidate will demonstrate that the management options for this condition can be
behavioural therapy, bladder retraining, changes in lifestyle, pharmacological treatment and
surgery.*

### Supportive treatment
Straightforward explanation of the condition to the patient is necessary.          1 mark
Behavioural therapy not only improves the patient's understanding of her
problem, but also provides effective relief of symptoms (60%) if the patient is
prepared to continue this at home.

Bladder retraining is useful in motivated patients. The patient is asked to delay     1 mark
micturition for increasing periods by suppressing the desire to void.

Fluid restriction if deemed necessary, avoiding stimulants such as tea, coffee        1 mark
and alcohol, and timed voiding may improve the symptoms.

Neuromodulation (S3 nerve stimulation via an electrode) may be tried in               1 mark
patients with no response to medical treatment who wish to avoid surgery.
Hypnosis and acupuncture are useful non-pharmacological treatments
providing up to 75% symptomatic relief in the short term.

### Medical treatment
Anticholinergics that can be used include oxybutynin, imipramine,                   2 marks
propantheline bromide, flavoxate and propiverine hydrochloride.
If the side effects are tolerable and the symptoms have improved, the
treatment can be continued indefinitely or it can be gradually tapered after
1 year. If symptoms do not improve in spite of the maximum tolerable dose,
then the treatment is changed to an alternative medication.

For patients using clean intermittent self-catheterization (CISC), intravesical       1 mark
oxybutynin provides the benefits with minimal side effects.
A number of new drugs, such as tropsium chloride, are in clinical trials and
should be available soon. They have better side-effect profiles.

### Surgical treatment
Cystodistension may help in minor degrees of detrusor instability, but it does         1 mark
not give long-term relief.

Clam ileocystoplasty provides up to 90% symptomatic relief, but it is a major          1 mark
operation fraught with complications.

The early complications include ileus, wound infection and bowel obstruction.    1 mark
Late complications could be repeated urinary tract infection, risk of neoplasm
and malabsorption.
The risk of postoperative voiding dysfunction requiring CISC is high
(40–100%).

## Suggested reading

Cardozo L. Detrusor instability, in RW Shaw, WP Soutter and SL Stanton (eds.)
    *Gynaecology*, 2nd edn. London: Churchill Livingstone; 1998. pp. 739–52.

4. A 50-year-old woman undergoes hysterectomy with bilateral oophorectomy for stage Ia poorly differentiated endometrial cancer. She wishes to
   commence on hormone replacement therapy (HRT). How will you counsel her regarding the pros and cons of HRT?

*The use of HRT in any woman should be discussed as far as the risks and benefits are con-
cerned, and then in the context of her condition. The possibility of oestrogen with progestogens HRT should be discussed in case of an oestrogen-sensitive tumour.*

Strong indications for starting HRT are very severe climacteric symptoms,           1 mark
sleep disturbances, severe atrophic urogenital changes, and high risk for
osteoporosis.

The long-term oestrogen therapy protects against osteoporosis.                      1 mark

It may protect against Alzheimer's disease, colon cancer, periodontal disease       1 mark
and cataracts.

The cardiovascular benefits are not yet definitely proven; prospective              1 mark
randomized controlled trials are still in progress.

HRT also favourably affects mood, libido and urinary symptoms.                      1 mark

The risks include increased incidence of breast cancer (increased from 45/1000     1 mark
to 47/1000 at the end of 5 years).

Slightly increased risk of venous thromboembolism (from 8 in 100 000 to 31          1 mark
in 100 000).
Perception of weight gain, although this is not linked directly to HRT.

With very early tumour, it is unlikely that there will be a recurrence with HRT.    1 mark
The patient is advised to report back in case of symptoms suggestive of
recurrence.

Progestogens given alone are not shown to be of much benefit, but combined          1 mark
progestogen and oestrogen HRT could be tried.
It is not known whether added progestogens will protect against recurrence of
endometrial adenocarcinoma.

If there is strong family history or personal history of breast cancer or           1 mark
thromboembolism, other alternatives such as tibolone or selective oestrogen
receptor modulators, e.g. raloxifene, can be tried.
Healthy lifestyle habits, such as weight-bearing exercise, reducing alcohol
intake, high-fibre diet and stopping smoking, are of benefit.

## Suggested reading

Creasman WT. Recommendations regarding estrogen replacement therapy after treatment of endometrial cancer. *Oncology* 1992; 6: 23–7.

Hillard T. Principles of hormone replacement therapy: part 1. *Trends in Urology, Gynaecology and Sexual Health* 2000; 5(5): 22–7.

5. Debate the proposition of introducing selective chlamydia screening in the UK.

*A good candidate will discuss the fact that chlamydia screening fulfils WHO criteria, and will state the risks and benefits of such a programme.*

Chlamydia is the most common, curable sexually transmitted infection in the Western world. It is an important problem. — 1 mark

Chlamydia infection is largely asymptomatic. — 1 mark
Numerous clinical conditions, including acute urethral syndrome, urethritis, mucopurulent cervicitis and prenatal infection, have been attributed to chlamydia trachomatis.
Up to 70% of infants delivered vaginally to women with chlamydia acquire the infection.

Untreated infection can have severe long-term consequences for women in the form of pelvic inflammatory disease (PID), infertility, ectopic pregnancy and chronic pelvic pain. — 1 mark

Evidence shows that screening for chlamydia can reduce the prevalence of chlamydia infection in women and the incidence of PID. — 1 mark
Its entire sequel, except for infertility, is preventable if it is treated in its asymptomatic phase.

The availability of DNA amplification tests with improved sensitivity and the introduction of single-dose therapy for the treatment of uncomplicated infection has eased the management of the infection. — 1 mark

The noninvasive testing is acceptable to the patients (urine and endocervical swab). — 1 mark
It is cost effective.

Selective screening is preferable to universal screening. The groups commonly targeted are: — 1 mark

- Everyone with symptoms of chlamydia infection
- All those attending genitourinary medicine clinics
- Women seeking termination of pregnancy
- Opportunistic screening of women under the age of 25 years and of women over 25 years with a new sexual partner or over two partners in the past year.

People with positive results might be looked upon as promiscuous. It can lead to feelings of guilt, unattractiveness and sexual dysfunction. — 1 mark

Screening women but not men can reduce further men's responsibility for   1 mark
sexual and reproductive health.

There will be additional monetary and time constraints on the GPs and family   1 mark
planning clinics that provide the screening.

## Suggested reading:

Duncan B, Hart G. Sexuality and health: the hidden costs for screening for chlamydia trachomatis. *BMJ* 1999; 318: 931–3.

Scottish Intercollegiate Network Guidelines. *Management of Genital Chlamydia Trachomatis Infection.* **http://www.show.scot.nhs.uk/sign/PDF/qrg42.pdf**.

# PAPER 9: OBSTETRICS

1. Discuss the potential harmful effects of vaginal delivery on the pelvic floor and the steps to reduce them.

2. An ultrasound scan performed following raised alphafetoprotein at 17 weeks gestation reveals an abdominal wall defect in the fetus. How will you counsel the parents?

3. Critically appraise the options of managing slow progress in the active phase of first stage in a primigravida who has spontaneous onset of labour at term.

4. A 30-year-old woman who has undergone renal transplantation 5 months ago is contemplating pregnancy. What preconceptual counselling will you offer her?

5. Justify your management of confirmed spontaneous rupture of the membranes at 28 weeks gestation in a previously normal pregnancy.

1. Discuss the potential harmful effects of vaginal delivery on the pelvic floor and the steps to reduce them.

*A good candidate will mention the important potential injuries to the pelvic floor from vaginal delivery, such as stress urinary incontinence, faecal incontinence and prolapse. Women with third- and fourth-degree tears have a higher incidence of problems. The majority of deliveries are unproblematic. Caesarean section helps to reduce the incidence of the above problems. Ventouse is less traumatic than forceps. Routine episiotomy is not associated with a better outcome.*

The majority of vaginal deliveries are not followed by problems to the pelvic floor.          1 mark
The damage is most likely to occur during the first vaginal delivery.

### Potential harmful effects of vaginal delivery
The incidence of genuine stress incontinence after vaginal delivery varies          1 mark
between 8 and 36%, depending on the time of delivery, and increases with the number of deliveries.
Women who have this problem antenatally are at higher risk postpartum, and this is presumed to be a hormonal effect rather than the effect of vaginal delivery.

Between 42 and 80% of women who deliver vaginally have partial pelvic floor          1 mark
denervation.
In the long term, combined with age this is likely to contribute to genital tract prolapse.

Vaginal delivery can damage the anal sphincter muscles. The incidence of          1 mark
faecal incontinence increases with the number of vaginal deliveries.
Third- and fourth-degree tears are associated with higher rate of faecal incontinence.

### Preventive strategies
Ventouse delivery causes less damage to maternal pelvic floor than forceps. So,          1 mark
if instrumental delivery is indicated, ventouse should be the instrument of first choice.

Difficult vaginal deliveries are avoided by using sound obstetric principles.          1 mark
Intensive pelvic floor exercises have no benefit in reducing the incidence of incontinence, although they do reduce the incidence of perineal pain after delivery.

Repair of fourth-degree tear by a senior obstetrician or surgeon has not shown          1 mark
to make a difference.
Accurate primary technique of suturing, however, prevents sphincter defects in some cases.

Whether a policy of restricted or liberal use of episiotomy is followed, the rates    1 mark
and severity of incontinence, dyspareunia and other problems are similar post-
delivery.

Occasionally, surgical revision of episiotomy scar (Fenton's operation) may be    1 mark
required.

Elective caesarean section may protect the pelvic floor from denervation    1 mark
injury, dyspareunia, faecal and urinary incontinence, but intrapartum
caesarean section may not.

## Suggested reading

Feldan GB, Freiman JA. Prophylactic caesarean section at term? *N Engl J Med* 1985;
    312: 1264–7.

Sultan AH, Kamm MA, Bartram CI, Hudson CN. Perineal damage at delivery.
    *Contemp Rev Obstet Gynaecol* 1994; 6(1): 18–24.

2. An ultrasound scan performed following raised alphafetoprotein at 17 weeks gestation reveals an abdominal wall defect in the fetus. How would you counsel the parents?

*A good candidate will structure the information into antenatal, intrapartum and postpartum.*

### Antenatal
Causes of raised alphafetoprotein should be explained to the parents: spina bifida, abdominal wall defects, bleeding, and more.     1 mark
Inform the parents of the differential diagnosis of abdominal wall defect, i.e. gastroschisis, omphalocele, simple hernia.

Other anomalies may be associated in case the anomaly looks like omphalocele, such as chromosomal or cardiac anomalies.     1 mark

Further investigations, such as fetal echocardiography and detailed ultrasound, need to be arranged.     1 mark

As omphalocele is associated with a 20% of aneuploidy, karyotyping is offered.     1 mark

Termination of pregnancy is an appropriate option before viability.     1 mark

Serial growth scans beyond 28 weeks are arranged as fetus with gastroschisis is at risk of intrauterine growth restriction and preterm labour.     1 mark

The prognosis of these potential complications should be mentioned briefly.     1 mark

Meeting with the neonatologist and the paediatric surgeons is arranged if the pregnancy is continued. They should discuss the outline of management once the baby is born.     1 mark
Information leaflets reinforce the counselling.

### Delivery
Vaginal delivery is usually appropriate.     1 mark
Caesarean section is reserved for obstetric indications or if the liver is extracorporeal.

### Postnatal
Risk of recurrence is low in most situations (<1%).     1 mark
Parents require a lot of psychological support in this stressful time.

## Suggested reading
Sermer M, Benzie R, Pitson L, *et al.* Prenatal diagnosis and management of congenital defects of the anterior abdominal wall. *Am J Obstet Gynecol* 1987; 156: 308–12.

3. Critically appraise the options of managing slow progress in the active phase of first stage in a primigravida who has spontaneous onset of labour at term.

---

*The candidate is expected to know how the diagnosis is reached. Conservative management: if maternal and fetal conditions are satisfactory, labour can be allowed to continue. Active management with artificial rupture of membranes (ARM), oxytocin, analgesia and reassessment is the alternative. There is no evidence in favour of either. Discussion with the parturient and taking her wishes into consideration is important.*

Slow progress in the active phase of first stage is diagnosed by poor rate of cervical dilatation, i.e.<1 cm/h in a primigravida.                              1 mark
Slow progress should alert one of the possibilities of abnormal labour, but should not automatically result in intervention.
Cephalopelvic disproportion and malpositions must be considered when progress is slow.

**Conservative**
The labour can be allowed to continue if the condition of the mother and the          1 mark
fetus is satisfactory.

The presence of a supportive companion and ambulation during labour has             1 mark
shown to result in shorter labours and less use of oxytocics.

**Medical (active)**
The active management of poor progress is a combination of:                          2 marks

- Artificial rupture of membranes (ARM): leads to reduction in the duration of labour by 60–120 min
- Intravenous oxytocin infusion with titration
- Adequate analgesia
- Reassessment at a fixed interval

(*allot ½ mark for each point mentioned*)

Injudicious use of oxytocin can lead to intrapartum fetal hypoxia. It is              1 mark
advisable to do continuous fetal monitoring if oxytocin infusion is commenced.

The use of early ARM and early use of oxytocin to shorten labour does not             1 mark
confer any specific benefit to mother or fetus.

Active management of labour reduces the duration of the first stage of labour         1 mark
(50–120 min) without affecting the rate of caesarean section and maternal
satisfaction.

Approximately half of the women deemed to have slow progress perform    1 mark
equally well regardless of whether active management is commenced.
It is appropriate to discuss the options with the patient and then manage
according to her wishes, because patient choice is an important issue.

**Surgical**
If after adequate trial of oxytocin there is no progress, caesarean section is    1 mark
required.

## Suggested reading

Fraser W, Vendittelli F, Krauss I, Breart G. Effects of early augmentation of labour
    with amniotomy and oxytocin in nulliparous women: a meta-analysis. *Br J Obstet
    Gynaecol* 1998; 105: 189–94.

Sadler LC, Davison T, LME McCowan. A randomised controlled trial and meta-
    analysis of active management of labour. *Br J Obstet Gynaecol* 2000; 107: 909–15.

4. A 30-year-old woman who has undergone renal transplantation 5 months ago is contemplating pregnancy. What counselling will you offer her?

*A good candidate will answer this question with the usual structure of the prognosis and issues specific to preconceptual, antenatal and intrapartum periods.*

## Preconceptual

It is advisable to wait 1–2 years after transplantation before embarking on a pregnancy.                                                              1 mark
This is because if renal function is normal for 2 years post-transplant, an improved 5-year transplant survival rate of about 80% can be anticipated.
Also, maintenance levels of immunosuppresive drugs will have been reached, thus minimizing any risk to the fetus.

Genetic counselling should be offered if the reason for renal failure was a familial disorder such as polycystic kidney disease or medullary sponge kidney.   1 mark

The other preconception advice, such as regular intake of 400 μg folic acid daily, avoiding smoking and alcohol, and having healthy diet, is not to be overlooked.   1 mark

## Antenatal

Steroids: the risk of teratogenic effects is very low.                         1 mark
Immunosuppressants: reported teratogenic problems are rare.

Antihypertensives: change from ACE inhibitors and pure beta blocker is advised.   1 mark
Antibiotics: continue, although a change of drug may be necessary.

There is an increased risk of pregnancy-induced hypertension, preterm delivery, intrauterine growth restriction (IUGR), urinary tract infection and graft rejection.   2 marks
(*allot ½ mark each for any four of the five risks*)

Pregnancy does not adversely affect long-term renal function.                  1 mark
Regular assessments of renal function (urea/creatinine/urate) are necessary.

There is an increased risk of early and late pregnancy loss. Regular assessment of fetal growth is necessary.   1 mark
The chance of a successful outcome is reduced to 70% if complications occur before 28 weeks.

## Delivery

A transplanted kidney does not obstruct labour.                                1 mark
Early delivery and caesarean section depend upon obstetric indications.

## Suggested reading

Nelson-Piercy C. Renal disease, in *Handbook of Obstetric Medicine*, 1st edn. Oxford: Isis Medical Media; 1997. pp. 155–8.

5. Justify your management of confirmed spontaneous rupture of the membranes at 28 weeks gestation in a previously normal pregnancy.

*A good candidate will demonstrate their awareness of risks of infection and preterm delivery, efficacy of potential treatments and risk/benefit of timing and route of delivery.*

## Conservative

At gestation less than 34 weeks, the objective is to prolong the pregnancy if there are no signs of fetal or maternal infection in order to minimize the risks associated with prematurity.                                                    1 mark

Tests for maternal well-being: serial monitoring of temperature, pulse, high vaginal swab and C-reactive protein.                                          2 marks

Vaginal examination is avoided unless the woman is in established labour, due to the increased risk of ascending infection.                                 1 mark

Periodic tests on the fetus: daily cardiotocography, twice-weekly biophysical profile, weekly liquor volume and Doppler studies, fortnightly growth scans.   2 marks

## Medical

Use of antibiotics: treatment of bacterial vaginosis with metronidazole or clindamycin, and of beta haemolytic streptococci with penicillin, is beneficial. Antibiotic treatment helps in increasing the interval to delivery and decreasing the risk of infection. However, there is no evidence to date that their use improves neonatal outcome.                                                  1 mark

A course of corticosteroids to induce fetal lung maturation is recommended. The data on repeated use are controversial.                                    1 mark

Use of tocolytic drugs such as nifedipine or ritodrine is recommended in case of threatened preterm labour until time is gained for action of steroids on the fetal lung (use of indomethacin is not desirable) or in utero transfer to a centre with neonatal care facilities.                                             1 mark

## Surgical

Timing of delivery and route: at any time, if signs of chorioamnionitis or fetal distress develop, it is necessary to deliver the fetus by the safest route possible, i.e. induction of labour or caesarean section.                            1 mark

## Suggested reading

Cararach V. Premature rupture of membranes: maternal and perinatal complications. *PACE Review No. 95/08.* London: RCOG Press; 1995.

Kenyon S, Boulvain M. Antibiotics for preterm premature rupture of membranes [Cochrane Review]. Cochrane Pregnancy and Childbirth Group, in The Cochrane Library, Issue 3, 2000. Oxford: Update software.

# PAPER 9: GYNAECOLOGY

1. Mention the potential urological consequences of hysterectomy, and describe how they may be avoided.

2. A 30-year-old woman who had an intrauterine contraception device IUCD fitted 16 months ago is referred by her GP because of non-visualization of the IUCD threads. Discuss the various options of management.

3. A 17-year-old girl is referred by her GP with severe crampy lower abdominal pains during her periods. Justify how you will approach this problem.

4. Debate the place of laparoscopic ovarian diathermy in the treatment of polycystic ovarian syndrome.

5. Critically appraise the role of surgery in epithelial ovarian cancer.

1. Mention the potential urological consequences of hysterectomy and describe how they may be avoided.

*A good candidate will be expected to write about the following complications and strategies for prevention: bladder – infection, hypotonia, fistula; ureters – early and late damage. An alternative way of structuring this answer is to divide it into preoperative, intraoperative and postoperative risks, and respective preventive steps.*

Removal of pelvic mass may reduce lower urinary tract symptoms. Minor postoperative symptoms are both transient and common.                          1 mark

**Urinary tract infection** is common. It is related to catheterization and stasis of urine.                                                                 1 mark

It is reduced by prophylactic antibiotics and keeping the duration of catheterization to a minimum. It is unlikely to represent a long-term problem.   1 mark

**Bladder damage** occurs in about 1 in 200 cases, and is more common after a previous caesarean section. Immediate damage occurs by sharp or blunt dissection, and later by avascular necrosis.                                    1 mark

Prevention: careful dissection, an empty bladder, use of subtotal hysterectomy, and the use of longer catheterization with difficult dissections or presence of haematuria and the recognition and repair of injuries when they occur.      1 mark

**Short-term voiding disorders** are due to pain, immobility and excess intravenous fluids. Longer-term disorders are due to nerve plexus damage with an increased incidence in radical surgery.                                     1 mark
Taking care of the causative factors and management of retention is adequate.

**Genuine stress incontinence and detrusor instability** are unlikely consequences, since the pelvic floor and pudendal nerves remain intact and any neurological damage would result in hypotonic rather than hypertonic detrusor activity.                                                            1 mark
Formation of urological fistulae is a rare complication of hysterectomy but needs appropriate management if diagnosed.

**Ureteric damage** occurs in about 1 in 500–1000 cases for benign disease and 1 in 100 in malignancy, and is even higher if preoperative radiotherapy is used. The rate is about 14 in 1000 laparoscopic hysterectomies.                    1 mark
Damage can be immediate (cutting, ligating) or late (avascular necrosis). Risk of damage is higher with distorted anatomy, e.g. endometriosis.

Prevention includes the surgeon's awareness of the risk of injury to the ureters throughout the entire pelvic dissection. It should be dissected sufficiently to   1 mark allow their identification and retraction out of harm's way. It can be reduced by judicious use of the subtotal operation.

When injury is recognized during the operation, repairing it with help of urologic surgeons is prudent.

1 mark

## Suggested reading

Petri E. Urological trauma in gynaecological surgery: diagnosis and management. *Curr Opin Obstet Gynecol* 1999; 11(5): 495–8.

2. A 30-year-old woman who had an intrauterine contraceptive device (IUCD) fitted 16 months ago is referred by her GP because of non-visualization of the threads. Discuss the various options of management.

*Lost threads may indicate expulsion, threads curled up in the uterus or cervical canal, or extrauterine device perforation. A good candidate will discuss the management in the light of each of these possibilities.*

### Investigation
If pregnancy cannot be excluded, or if the device is not felt, an ultrasound scan is the ideal investigation.                                                                  1 mark

If pregnancy is excluded and the IUCD is not in the uterus, it is appropriate to arrange for X-rays in the first 10 days of the cycle with a uterine sound *in situ.*                1 mark

### Conservative
Threads may be difficult to see and feel. Good light, proper speculum and cleaning of cervix may be necessary sometimes before the threads are visualized.                                                                              1 mark

If the IUCD is placed centrally in the uterus, then reassure the patient and offer the alternative to leave the IUCD *in situ* and scan yearly or remove and reinsert new IUCD.                                                              1 mark

### Medical
Artery forceps in the cervical canal may locate the thread. If the IUCD is in the cervical canal, remove it and reinsert a new one. When the patient wishes the IUCD to be removed, there are varioustechniques for bringing down threads (using Emmet's thread retriever or Helix). If that is unsuccessful, a blunt-ended hook may be used.                                                      1 mark

If the IUCD is not seen in the peritoneal cavity, assume spontaneous expulsion and offer to refit the IUCD.                                                           1 mark

### Surgical
The removal of the device under hysteroscopic control is indicated if it is not possible to get it out easily in the clinic and the device is intrauterine.              1 mark

If a device is extrauterine, it needs to be removed under laparoscopic guidance as the copper produces a sterile inflammatory reaction with adhesions.                  1 mark

If a pregnancy has occurred and the patient decides to continue with it, it is important to ensure that the device is not left after the pregnancy. The patient should be advised to check on this postpartum. If necessary a scan and/or X-ray should be performed.

1 mark

If the intrauterine pregnancy is not wanted, discuss early termination and then arrange investigations for the missing IUCD.

1 mark

3. A 17-year-old girl is referred by her GP with severe crampy lower abdominal pains during her periods. Justify how you will approach this problem.

*The clinical approach should be systematic: history, examination, investigations and treatment (supportive, medical and surgical).*

### History

Detailed history of onset, duration and type of pain and other associated symptoms, along with the details of menstrual history.                              1 mark
The chance should be taken to explore her family and social background, and to find out how much this dysmenorrhoea affects her daily routine.

### Examination

Abdominal examination is done. If the girl is not a virgo intacta, a pelvic examination is carried out, but this is rarely useful.                              1 mark

### Investigations

Ultrasound scan is occasionally useful if pathology is suspected.                   1 mark
In any teenage girl in whom standard treatment fails, it is important to rule out uterine anomaly, particularly rudimentary uterine horns, by means of imaging.

### Supportive treatment

The diagnosis in the majority of cases is primary dysmenorrhoea, and the explanation of its physiological basis given sympathetically is reassuring to most girls.                              1 mark

### Medical treatment

Simple painkillers such as aspirin and codeine can be tried.                        1 mark

As the pain is due to release of prostaglandins, fenamates such as mefenamic acid or propionic acid derivatives (flurbiprofen) are very effective for symptomatic relief in 80% of patients.                              1 mark

Oral contraceptive pills inhibit ovulation and relieve dysmenorrhoea. They have other obvious advantages, such as reduction in the amount of bleeding, and are a first-line treatment if the girl wishes contraception as well.                              1 mark

For spasms, antispasmodic drugs such as dicyclomine butylbromide have been tried empirically, but they have no proven benefit.                              1 mark
Other features associated with primary dysmenorrhoea such as vomiting rarely require treatment with antiemetics once the primary problem is taken care of.

### Surgery

Surgical therapy (e.g. forced cervical dilation or presacral neurectomy) is not considered appropriate in this condition.                              1 mark

Laparoscopy is indicated only in cases of resistant dysmenorrhoea, as disorders    1 mark
such as endometriosis and pelvic inflammatory disease need to be ruled out.
The value of laparoscopic uterine nerve ablation is not fully established.

## Suggested reading

Muse KN. Menstrual cycle disorders. *Obstet Gynecol Clin North Am* 1990: 430–1.

4. Debate the place of laparoscopic ovarian diathermy in the treatment of polycystic ovarian syndrome.

*A good candidate will indicate that laparoscopic ovarian drilling is the surgical treatment of choice for infertility in the case of polycystic ovaries. The pros and cons of this treatment should be discussed.*

**Pros**

Laparoscopic ovarian diathermy (LOD) is the surgical treatment of choice in women suffering from infertility due to polycystic ovarian syndrome (PCOS) resistant to clomiphene.                                                    1 mark

The risk of multiple pregnancy is low, hence its sequels (i.e. greater monitoring, problems with prenatal screening, pregnancy-induced hypertension, antepartum haemorrhage, preterm labour and financial implications) are avoided.                                                     1 mark

The risk of ovarian hyperstimulation is removed.                        1 mark
It is more cost effective than gonadotrophin treatment.

Once-only treatment.                                                    1 mark
No intensive monitoring required.
It can be done at the same time as laparoscopic pelvic assessment in women who fail to conceive after a trial of clomiphene therapy.

Its role in primary treatment of PCOS is not yet determined.            1 mark
As a secondary treatment for clomiphene-resistant PCOS, there are insufficient data available to determine efficacy of LOD in terms of ovulation and pregnancy rates over gonadotrophins.

A 12-month cumulative pregnancy rate of 54–84% has been reported in        1 mark
patients with no other abnormality.
It reduces serum LH levels, thereby reducing the subsequent miscarriage rate after conception.

**Cons**
There is no consensus at present over the right dose of diathermy.        1 mark
None of the techniques of drilling (diathermy v. laser, unilateral v. bilateral ovarian drilling) have proven advantages over each other.

There is uncertainty regarding the degree of permanent damage done by the   1 mark
treatment. There have been a few cases of ovarian failure post-procedure reported in the literature.

The duration of effect is 6–12 months, hence it is not done for other symptoms of PCOS such as acne or hirsutism.
The potential complications and risks of anaesthetic and laparoscopy exist.

1 mark

The risk of periovarian adhesions and further reduction in fertility rate exists. This can be reduced by abdominal lavage and early second-look laparoscopy and adhesiolysis if necessary.

1 mark

## Suggested reading

Farquhar C, Vanderkerchkhove P, Arnot M and Lilford R. Laparoscopic 'drilling' by diathermy or laser for ovulation induction in anovulatory polysystic ovary syndrome [review]. The Cochrane Library, Issue 2, 2000. Oxford: Update software.

5. Critically appraise the role of surgery in epithelial ovarian cancer.

*A good candidate will discuss the pros and cons of staging laparotomy, debulking surgery, second-look surgery, interval debulking and palliative surgery.*

**Staging laparotomy** done for epithelial ovarian cancer (EOC) is important:          1 mark

- To decide subsequent mode of management (whether adjunctive chemotherapy is required in early disease )
- As a prognostic indicator for an individual
- For providing meaningful data for clinical trials

Federation of International Gynaecologists and Obstetricians (FIGO) staging refers to total abdominal hysterectomy, bilateral salpingo-oophorectomy, infracolic omentectomy with ascitic fluid cytology and retroperitoneal lymph node sampling.

**Debulking surgery**
**Pros**                                                                                    2 marks
Better response to subsequent treatment in the form of chemotherapy or radiotherapy.
Treatment or prevention of complications caused by tumour mass (bowel obstruction, ascites).
Improved quality of life – psychological benefits, enhanced immunological competence.
(Allot 1 mark each for any 2 of the above 3 points.)

**Cons**
Aggressive surgical excision of tumour is not without risks and sequel, which          1 mark
may sometimes adversely affect survival and quality of life.

Residual tumour size is a major determinant in the survival.                            1 mark
Prognosis is better if operated by gynaecological oncologist rather than
a general surgeon.

The usefulness of these surgeries at improving survival rates is not proven.            1 mark

**Conservative surgery** in stage Ia disease in the form of unilateral salpingo-       1 mark
oophorectomy with staging laparotomy is appropriate if the patient is keen on
retaining fertility.

**Interval debulking surgery** is performed half way through chemotherapy             1 mark
cycle, when response to chemotherapy is identifiable.
Pros: evidence suggests 33% reduction in risk of death.
Cons: The cost–benefit implications are unknown. The additional survival
time of 6 months might be spent in recovering from a major surgery, and the
value is questionable.

**Second-look laparoscopy or laparotomy** have no proven benefits other than     1 mark
when done as a palliative procedure. Hence they should be done only in the
context of clinical trial.

**Palliative surgery**, such as resection, bypass or colostomy, improves the quality     1 mark
of life and alleviates symptoms, but survival is unaffected.

## Suggested reading

Kehoe S. The value of surgery in ovarian cancer. *The Obstetrician and Gynaecologist* 2000; 2(3): 5–8.

Soutter P. The role of surgery in ovarian cancer. *CME Self-Assessment Review No. 97/10*. London: RCOG Press; 1997.

# Paper 10: OBSTETRICS

1. A 30-year-old woman who has ileostomy due to Crohn's disease wishes to start her family. Give an account of your counselling of this patient in the prepregnancy clinic.

2. Summarize the options in managing a multiparous woman who has been found to have unstable lie at 38 weeks gestation.

3. A 40-year-old woman who is pregnant after *in vitro* fertilization (IVF) requests amniocentesis of her twin pregnancy. One fetus is found to have Down's syndrome. Discuss the issues involved.

4. Discuss the potential complications and your management of hyperemesis gravidarum in a primigravida at 14 weeks gestation.

5. A healthy 37-year-old primigravida presents with a singleton pregnancy in cephalic presentation and engaged presenting part at 38 weeks gestation. She requests an elective caesarean section. The pregnancy has been uneventful so far. Justify your approach.

1. A 30-year old-woman who has ileostomy due to Crohn's disease wishes to start her family. Give an account of your counselling of this patient in the prepregnancy clinic.

*A good candidate will structure the answer into preconceptual, antenatal, intrapartum and postpartum advice.*

### Preconceptual
In general, pregnancy has no effect on the course of the disease.     1 mark
Most women with prior surgery tolerate the pregnancy well.

The woman should try to conceive during periods of disease remission to     1 mark
reduce the risk of miscarriage.

Fertility is normal in well-controlled disease.     1 mark
Periconceptual folic acid is advisable, as for any other woman planning
pregnancy.

### Antenatal
Crohn's disease remains quiescent in about 75% of pregnant women.     1 mark
Exacerbation of the inactive Crohn's disease mostly occurs during the first
trimester.

Active disease during the course of pregnancy is associated with an increased     1 mark
rate of prematurity.

Some pregnant women with ileostomy or massive gut resection may develop     1 mark
problems, such as malabsorption of fat, fat-soluble vitamins and vitamin B12,
water and electrolyte imbalance, hyperoxaluria and cholelithiasis.

The management of acute attacks and chronic disease is not affected     1 mark
substantially by pregnancy.
The safety of metronidazole and azathioprine in early pregnancy is not proven.

### Delivery
Most women with quiescent disease and stoma have full-term normal     1 mark
deliveries.
Caesarean section is required only for obstetric indications and in women with
perianal Crohn's disease and abscesses.

### Postpartum
Postpartum flare may occur. Sulphasalazine and corticosteroids may be used     1 mark
safely throughout pregnancy and while breastfeeding.

Oral contraceptives are avoided for contraception as they might exacerbate the    1 mark
disease. Barrier or intrauterine contraceptives are recommended.

## Suggested reading

Nelson Piercy C. Gastrointestinal disease, in *Handbook of Obstetric Medicine*, 1st edn.
Oxford: Isis Medical Media; 1998. pp. 186–9.

2. Summarize the options in managing a multiparous woman who has been found to have unstable lie at 38 weeks gestation.

*A good candidate should structure the answer in a systematic clinical approach of history, examination, investigations, expectant and active management. Note that the question does not specify whether the woman is in labour.*

### History and examination
History checked carefully: family or personal history of diabetes mellitus should be checked.                                                    1 mark
Polyhydramnios should be ruled out by abdominal palpation.

A pelvic examination to identify any factor causing obstruction in the pelvis (e.g. tumour, fibroid) and to assess the Bishop's score. It is deferred in case of placenta praevia.                                                    1 mark

### Investigations
Real-time ultrasound is organized to identify significant malformations, polyhydramnios or pelvic tumours, and to localize placenta.                                                    1 mark

### Management
Prenatal options are between expectant and active management.
**Supportive**                                                    1 mark
No specific action is taken in the anticipation that the lie will become longitudinal before the membranes rupture or labour starts (happens in 80% of cases).
Admission may be advised due to the risk of cord prolapse in cases of spontaneous rupture of membranes. Midwives advise knee–elbow position.

When the membranes rupture or labour begins and the lie is longitudinal, the management of labour is as per normal after exclusion of cord presentation/ prolapse.                                                    1 mark
**Medical**
**Stabilizing induction**: external cephalic version (ECV) is performed on the delivery suite and after regular abdominal palpation to confirm that the longitudinal lie is maintained; intravenous oxytocin infusion is commenced and titrated to achieve regular uterine contractions.                                                    1 mark

Amniotomy is then performed. High amniotomy reduces the incidence of cord prolapse but is rarely done in modern obstetrics.                                                    1 mark

### Surgical
**Elective caesarean section**: at 38–39 weeks, an elective caesarean section can be carried out, ideally after converting the lie to longitudinal at laparotomy.                                                    1 mark

Indications: if ECV is contraindicated or failed, if there is a mechanical                    1 mark
obstruction to vaginal delivery, or if patient wishes it.

If the woman is in labour, external cephalic version or caesarean section are the    1 mark
options.

## Suggested reading

Mackenzie IZ. Unstable lie, in *High Risk Pregnancy Management Options*, DK James,
PJ Steer, CP Weiner and B Gonick (eds) 2nd edn. London: WB Saunders 1999.
pp. 199–205.

3. A 40-year-old woman who is pregnant after *in vitro* fertilization (IVF) requests amniocentesis of her twin pregnancy. One fetus is found to have Down's syndrome. Discuss the issues involved.

*A good candidate will discuss the options of conservative management and selective termination of the affected fetus. Termination of the twin pregnancy is unlikely to be acceptable in a couple conceived by IVF. It is important to differentiate mono- and dichorionic twins.*

### Counselling

Careful prior discussion and counselling in a tertiary referral centre with expertise in fetal medicine.                                                        1 mark

Offer the options:
Do nothing.                                                                      1 mark

Selective termination (ST).                                                      1 mark
Termination of pregnancy may not be acceptable to majority of parents.

Monoamniotic twins are a contraindication to ST.                                 1 mark

If the parents choose ST, reassure that although the experience is small, ST is mostly associated with term delivery of a healthy neonate (90%). Psychological support is often a neglected area of the care.                                    1 mark

Technique involves careful identification of the abnormal twin and intracardiac injection of potassium chloride.                                   1 mark
The complications, such as bleeding, ruptured membranes and loss of co-twin, is less (5–10%) if ST is done before 16 weeks gestation.                        1 mark

In monochorionic gestation, alternative techniques such as unipolar diathermy to the umbilical vessels or endoscopic ligation to the umbilical cord are required because of the risk of feto-fetal transfusion and ischaemic brain damage.                                                                         1 mark

Only experienced operators should perform ST.                                    1 mark

If the other twin survives in a monochorionic twin pregnancy:                     1 mark

- Monitor maternal platelets and clotting
- Monitor fetal growth and well being

## Suggested reading

Evans MI, Littman L, Isada NB, Johnson MP. Multifetal pregnancy reduction and selective termination, in DK James, PJ Steer, CP Weiner and B Gonick (eds). *High Risk Pregnancy Management Options*, 2nd edn. London: WB Saunders; 1999. pp. 1027–8.

4. Discuss the potential complications and your management of hyperemesis gravidarum in a primigravida at 14 weeks gestation.

---

*Enumerate the possible maternal and fetal complications. Supportive, medical and surgical
treatments should then be discussed.*

**Potential complications**
Adverse fetal outcome is unlikely unless very severe hyperemesis.                    1 mark

The potential maternal complications that can occur with severe hyperemesis           1 mark
are Mallory–Weiss syndrome and hepatorenal failure.

**History**: it is a diagnosis of exclusion.                                          1 mark
**Clinical examination** for hydration status and to rule out other pathology that
can cause similar symptoms (pyelonephritis, appendicitis, thyrotoxicosis,
gastroenteritis).

**Investigations**
Full blood count for haematocrit and white cell count.                               1 mark
Serum urea and electrolytes.
Liver function and thyroid function tests in resistant cases.
Urinalysis to exclude urinary tract infection.

Ultrasonography to rule out molar and twin pregnancy.                                 1 mark

**Supportive**
Nil by mouth until vomiting controlled.                                              1 mark
Intravenous fluid and electrolyte administration.
Psychological support.

**Medical**
Antiemetics reduce the nausea and vomiting in early pregnancy. The little            1 mark
information available on fetal outcome is reassuring.
Vitamin supplements: pyridoxine (vitamin B6) appears to be more effective in
reducing the severity of nausea. Thiamine is given to treat Wernicke's
encephalopathy.

Corticosteroids: short course of steroids has been shown to be useful in some        1 mark
studies in patients requiring hospitalization for hyperemesis.
Adrenocorticotropic hormone to treat hyperemesis gravidarum is not
beneficial.

Ginger and acupressure may be of benefit, but the evidence so far is weak.           1 mark
Antacids and H$_2$ receptor antagonists are administered to prevent acid peptic
disease.

**Surgical**

Total parenteral nutrition may be necessary if there is no response to the          1 mark
antiemetics and patient has lost more than 10% of body weight.

Termination of pregnancy may occasionally be necessary in uncontrollable
cases causing hepatorenal failure.

## Suggested reading

Jewell, D. Young, G. Interventions for nausea and vomiting in early pregnancy. [systematic review], Cochrane Pregnancy and Childbirth Group, in The Cochrane Library, Issue 3, 2000. Oxford: Update software.

5. A healthy 37-year-old primigravida presents with a singleton pregnancy in cephalic presentation and engaged presenting part at 38 weeks gestation. She requests an elective caesarean section. The pregnancy has been uneventful so far. Justify your approach.

*A good candidate should discuss the risks and benefits of caesarean section and allow the woman to make an 'informed decision'.*

**Risks**

The risk of maternal mortality following caesarean section is three times higher than spontaneous vaginal delivery.                          1 mark

Maternal morbidity is higher: infection, haemorrhage, anaesthesia, higher repeat caesarean section rate.                                      1 mark

Delayed recovery.                                                          1 mark
Prolonged hospital stay.
Increased requirement for analgesia.
Increased demand on resources.

Higher risk of respiratory morbidity in neonates (transient tachypnoea of newborn) when performed before the expected due dates.              1 mark

**Benefits**

Reduced risk of stress incontinence, bowel incontinence, perineal pain, dyspareunia, prolapse.                                              2 marks
(*allot 2 marks for mentioning any four out of the above*)

Convenience and choice.                                                    1 mark
It is better than having an emergency caesarean section or a difficult instrumental vaginal delivery.

Reduced neonatal mortality (1 in 90 000 in elective caesarean section v. 1 in 1000 in vaginal delivery) and risk of injury.                         1 mark

**Informed decision**

The woman's concerns and anxieties should be noted and her doubts cleared.   1 mark
The decision should be a joint enterprise by patient and clinician.

We should respect the woman's view and choice if it is fully informed, if she  1 mark
expresses a logical reason for wanting a caesarean section, and if she can demonstrate an understanding of the risks of the procedure. This needs to be documented properly.

## Suggested reading

Paterson SB. Should doctors perform an elective caesarean section on request? *BMJ* 1998; 317: 462–5.

# PAPER 10: GYNAECOLOGY

1. A 49-year-old woman attends your clinic with a request for coil change. She has had a copper intrauterine contraceptive device (IUCD) *in situ* for the last 3 years. How will you advise her?

2. Debate the controversy in the management of a woman with a single smear showing mild dyskaryosis.

3. Discuss the presentation and management of severe ovarian hyperstimulation.

4. Give a brief account of the morbidity associated with chemotherapy for epithelial ovarian cancers. Discuss the steps that can be taken to reduce the side effects.

5. Discuss the measures that can optimize outcome related to the abdominal incisions in gynaecological surgery.

1. A 49-year-old woman attends your clinic with a request for coil change. She has had a copper intrauterine contraceptive device (IUCD) *in situ* for the last 3 years. How will you advise her?

*A good candidate will demonstrate the knowledge that fertility declines with age and there is no need for this woman to change coil. This opportunity is also taken to ensure her general well-being, screening status and hormone replacement.*

Explain to the woman that fertility decreases rapidly with age.                    1 mark

There is no necessity for change of coil or its removal until 1 year after                    2 marks
menopause.

Replacement of the IUCD is associated with increased chances of failure in the                    1 mark
first few months.

Enquire about menstrual pattern and associated problems.                    1 mark

If menorrhagia is a problem, fitting of Mirena intrauterine system after ruling                    1 mark
out pathology is an option.

This visit also provides an opportunity to ask about cervical smear screening                    1 mark
and breast self-examination.

The patient's awareness of menopausal symptoms can be gauged. Hormone                    1 mark
replacement therapy (HRT) and healthy lifestyle habits can be discussed.
If there are contraindications to HRT, alternative therapies can be discussed.

This information should be backed up by information leaflets, videotapes and                    1 mark
support groups.

Commencing HRT before cessation of periods may make it difficult to decide                    1 mark
when to remove the device and discontinue contraception. In such a case, it is
probably appropriate to leave IUCD *in situ* until the age of 55 years.

2. Debate the controversy in the management of a woman with a single smear showing mild dyskaryosis.

*A good candidate will demonstrate that contrary to the current guidelines from the NHS Cervical Screening Programme (repeat smear in 6 months and if abnormal refer for colposcopy), many experts believe that immediate referral and selective treatment is the optimal strategy. The pros and cons of both policies should be discussed.*

The controversy surrounding the approach to mild dyskaryosis regards the problem of whether cytological surveillance or immediate referral for colposcopy is the optimal management.                                          1 mark

According to the National Health Service Cervical Screening Programme (NHS CSP), the protocol for management of mild dyskaryosis states:

1. Repeat the smear in 6 months                                        1 mark
2. If normal, repeat after another 6 months; if persistently normal, return to normal recall

3. If abnormal again, refer for colposcopy.                            1 mark

Many experts recommend immediate referral for colposcopy and a select-and-    1 mark
treat management strategy of all women with any degree of dyskaryosis.

**Benefits of immediate referral**
About 20% of these women will have underlying cervical intraepithelial        1 mark
neoplasia (CIN) grade III that will be treated.

A policy of cytological surveillance allows an opportunity for default of      1 mark
women who are at an increased risk of invasive cancer. This is probably
reduced by immediate referral.
50% of these women do not revert to cytological normality and will eventually
be referred for colposcopy.

A policy of immediate referral to colposcopy may be financially less expensive 1 mark
in the long term according to some studies on cost–benefit analysis.
Women generally prefer active management due to anxiety associated with an
abnormal smear.

**Risks of immediate referral**
Half of these women will have normal smear on repeat and will not need         1 mark
colposcopy.

Increase in waiting times for colposcopy: 5% of women who have smears will       1 mark
be diagnosed to have mild dyskaryosis, translating into 250 000 additional
women having colposcopy annually.
Increased immediate demand on funds.

Increased risk of intervention and overtreatment and adverse psychological        1 mark
impact on the women.
Although up to 20% of women with low-grade lesions will develop CIN III,
many studies have shown that early colposcopy has not reduced the incidence
of invasive carcinoma.

## Suggested reading

Flannelly G, Kitchener H. Every woman with an abnormal cervical smear should be
referred for treatment: debate. *Clin Obstet Gynecol* 1995; 38(3): 585–91.

Shafi MI, Luesley DM, Jordan JA, Dunn JA, *et al.* Randomised trial of immediate versus deferred treatment strategies for the management of minor cervical cytological abnormalities. *Br J Obstet Gynaecol* 1997; 104(5): 590–4.

3. Discuss the presentation and management of severe ovarian hyperstimulation.

*A good candidate will exhibit the knowledge answer that severe ovarian hyperstimulation syndrome (OHSS) is life threatening. Management of severe OHSS should be summarized.*

### History and examination
Symptoms are those of hypovolaemia, hyponatraemia and effusions.                    1 mark

Signs of severe OHSS include clinical ascites, hydrothorax,                          2 marks
haemoconcentration (haematocrit >45% and white cell count >15 000/ml),
oliguria with normal serum creatinine, liver dysfunction, ovarian size usually>
12 cm.
Hospitalization is required.

### Investigations                                                                   1 mark
Full blood count and haematocrit.
Liver function tests.
Urea, electrolytes, creatinine.
Coagulation profile.

Ultrasound scan of abdomen, pelvis.                                                  1 mark
Chest X-ray or scan to rule out pleural effusion.

### Supportive treatment                                                             3 marks
Monitoring of vital signs and urine output.
Admission to intensive care unit may be required.
Thromboembolic deterrent stockings.
Correction of fluid balance: intravenous fluids (albumin if necessary).
Appropriate liaison with the centre initiating treatment if the patient presents
to the nearest hospital.
Psychological support.
(*allot ½ mark for each point*)

### Medical treatment                                                                1 mark
Heparin for thromboprophylaxis.
Adequate analgesia: paracetamol, codeine, opiates.

### Surgical treatment                                                               1 mark
Drainage of effusions for symptomatic relief.
Rarely laparotomy if ovarian torsion suspected to relieve the torsion, but this
should be undertaken with caution.
In exceptional circumstances, termination of pregnancy may be required as a
life-saving procedure.

## Suggested reading

Jenkins J, Mathur R. Ovarian hyperstimulation syndrome (PACE). *CME Self-Assessment Review No. 98/06.* London: RCOG Press; 1998.

4. Give a brief account of the morbidity associated with chemotherapy for epithelial ovarian cancers. Discuss the steps that can be taken to reduce the side effects.

*A good candidate will demonstrate that planning treatment on baseline blood count, renal and liver function tests, and ECG is important. Marks will only be given if the steps to minimize the side effects are written. Do not forget to compare and contrast cisplatin and carboplatin regarding their side effects.*

**General side effects** include nausea, vomiting, risk of leukaemia, bone marrow suppression (neutropenia, thrombocytopenia, anaemia) and its sequelae.

1 mark

**Specific side effects**

2 marks

Alkylating agents such as cyclophosphamide: alopecia, pulmonary fibrosis.
Cisplatin: ototoxicity, peripheral neuropathy, acute tubular necrosis.
Adriamycin: cardiomyopathy.
Paclitaxel: allergic reactions, cardiac arrhythmias.
(*allot ½ mark for each drug*)

**Steps to minimize side effects**
**Pretreatment**
Specialized treatment for cancer patients should be given in regional cancer centres.

1 mark

Perform baseline tests, i.e. full blood count, renal and liver function tests, electrocardiogram (ECG) to detect system dysfunction, and avoid drugs that will worsen the already existing compromise. These tests can also be used to monitor the toxicity.

1 mark

Alopecia is prevented by appropriate selection of chemotherapy; other methods of prevention are not of proven value. Cosmetic wigs should be supplied to patients who do have alopecia.
Paclitaxel and adriamycin are avoided in patients with heart disease.

1 mark

**During treatment**
Sedation, steroids, $H_2$ antagonists, and powerful antiemetics such as ondansetron before and during treatment help control the nausea and vomiting.

1 mark

Aggressive hydration and forced diuresis are required for nephrotoxic agents such as cisplatin.
Carboplatin is significantly less nephrotoxic, has no neurotoxic or ototoxic effects, and is used as a first-line therapy. Thrombocytopoenia is its dose-limiting toxicity, which needs to be monitored.

1 mark

**Post-treatment**
If a patient experiences prolonged myelosuppression (beyond 21 days after          1 mark
treatment), reduction of dose may be necessary.
In the event of fever, hospitalization and treatment with broad-spectrum
antibiotics that cover *Pseudomonas* is mandatory.

To limit the risk of leukaemia:                                                     1 mark

- Discontinue treatment if there is no response after three cycles
- Do not continue treatment beyond 1 year when it is no longer useful

## Suggested reading

Clarke-Pearson DL, Hurteau JA, Elbendary AA, Carney M. Chemotherapy of gyne-
cologic malignancies, in JA Rock and JD Thompson (eds). *Te Linde's Operative
Gynecology*, 8th edn. Philadelphia: Lippincot-Raven 1997. pp. 1607–34.

5. Discuss the measures that can optimize outcome related to the abdominal incisions in gynaecological surgery.

*A good candidate will discuss preoperative steps (advising regarding reducing smoking, chest physiotherapy), along with intraoperative measures to reduce the risk of infection, haematoma, pain, dehiscence and adhesions and to improve cosmesis.*

**Preoperative**
Ensure the patient's fitness for surgery.                                                                 1 mark
Improve preoperative general condition to reduce postoperative stress on the wound, e.g. reduction or cessation of smoking, chest physiotherapy.

**Intraoperative**
The site and extent of the incision should be requisite with the indication of    1 mark
operation. It could be transverse, oblique or vertical.

Midline longitudinal incisions allow more adequate access, especially in           1 mark
oncological surgery and in a patient with large pelvic mass, adhesions and endometriosis.

Cautery should be avoided on the skin to reduce the wound infection rate.          1 mark

Prophylactic single dose of a broad-spectrum antibiotic at induction halves the    1 mark
risk of postoperative infection.

Transverse suprapubic incisions have cosmetic advantages and cause less            1 mark
postoperative discomfort.
A subcuticular suture increases these benefits.

The likelihood of wound dehiscence and incisional hernia is higher in midline      1 mark
longitudinal incision.
Mass closure and use of nonabsorbable sutures reduce this risk.

Peritoneal closure has no benefits. On the contrary, it may increase the risk of   1 mark
intestinal obstruction resulting from adhesions.

The risk of postoperative wound infection can be reduced by strict aseptic         1 mark
precautions, careful haemostasis, and limiting wound contamination.

Wound drains minimize the risk of wound haematoma; this is particularly            1 mark
useful in women who are given prophylactic anticoagulant therapy.

# Part Three

# Mock Examinations

# PAPER 1: PRACTICE QUESTIONS

## OBSTETRICS

1. "The advantages of epidural analgesia in labour outweigh its disadvantages." Debate this statement.

2. Discuss the management of pregnancy and delivery in a 23-year-old primigravida who is seen in the antenatal clinic at 11 weeks of pregnancy with a history of congenital aortic stenosis.

3. What are the salient features in the management of vascular embolism associated with pregnancy?

4. Discuss the options for screening for chromosomal abnormalities in the first trimester of pregnancy.

5. What complications of caesarean section may occur within the first 2 weeks of puerperium? How may they be prevented?

## GYNAECOLOGY

1. Discuss the causes and management of dyspareunia in a lady of reproductive age group.

2. Describe the complications of irradiation for female genital cancer. How may these be treated?

3. A mother brings her daughter aged 7 years to consult you because of vaginal discharge. Discuss the investigation and management of this problem.

4. Discuss post-pill amenorrhoea and its management.

5. What aspects of management affect the outcome in *in vitro* fertilization (IVF)?

# PAPER 2: PRACTICE QUESTIONS

## OBSTETRICS

1. A 35-year-old multiparous woman presents with acute upper abdominal pain at 34 weeks gestation. Discuss the clinical approach in her management.

2. Critically appraise the value of the investigations performed in every pregnant woman as part of standard antenatal care.

3. How will you counsel a 36-year-old pregnant woman who is found to have choroid plexus cyst on her mid-trimester scan?

4. Discuss the management of a pregnant woman referred by her GP at 24 weeks gestation with blood pressure of 160/100 and +++ proteinuria.

5. Debate the medicolegal issues involved in intrapartum electronic fetal monitoring.

## GYNAECOLOGY

1. What are the possible immediate and remote complications of vaginal hysterectomy? Discuss steps to minimize them.

2. What factors affect the prognosis in a patient with gestational trophoblastic tumour?

3. Discuss the investigations for male factor infertility.

4. "Gynaecological day case surgery is good for both patient and the hospital." Debate this statement.

5. Evaluate the non-contraceptive benefits associated with oral contraceptive pills.

# **PAPER 3**: PRACTICE QUESTIONS

## OBSTETRICS

1. What is your clinical approach to a parturient who is diagnosed to have secondary arrest in labour?

2. Justify your management of a pregnant lady who presents with a painless vaginal bleed at 30 weeks gestation.

3. A primigravid woman with severe pre-eclampsia has an eclamptic fit during induction of labour by prostaglandins. Outline your management following this event.

4. Debate the means available to assess fetal well-being *in utero*.

5. Discuss the different options for diagnosing fetal anomaly in a twin pregnancy.

## GYNAECOLOGY

1. You have delivered a baby with ambiguous genitalia. How is this problem managed?

2. Critically evaluate the surgical procedures used in the management of stress incontinence of urine.

3. Discuss the place of tubal surgery in the management of infertility.

4. Evaluate the management of microinvasive carcinoma of the cervix in a woman of reproductive age group.

5. Discuss the role of progesterone in contraception.

# PAPER 4: PRACTICE QUESTIONS

## OBSTETRICS

1. Discuss the ways in which obstetric practice may reduce the incidence of brain damage in the newborn.

2. "Ultrasound scanning has removed the need for maternal serum screening." Debate this statement.

3. Discuss the management of a primigravida at 30 weeks gestation sent to the consultant clinic by a community midwife as "small for dates".

4. What are the issues you will discuss in the prepregnancy counselling of a 27-year-old woman whose father suffers from haemophilia A?

5. A 20-year-old woman who delivered 5 days ago is reported by the midwife as not caring for her baby or showing any interest in things around her. What are the psychiatric conditions she could be suffering from, and what is the optimal management?

## GYNAECOLOGY

1. Outline optimal management of a 1-cm vulval squamous carcinoma diagnosed in a 55-year-old woman.

2. A 28-year-old woman who has been trying to conceive for 2 years is diagnosed to have mild endometriosis on laparoscopy. What are her management options?

3. A 20-year-old university student who weighs 110 kg and has had one termination of pregnancy in the past attends for contraceptive advice. Counsel her.

4. Discuss steps to minimize complications in hysteroscopic surgery.

5. A nulliparous 20-year-old woman is referred to the gynaecology outpatient clinic as she has periods only when she is on the combined oral contraceptive pill. She is diagnosed to have premature ovarian failure. How will you counsel her?

# PAPER 5: PRACTICE QUESTIONS

## OBSTETRICS

1. What is the importance of establishing chorionicity in a twin pregnancy?

2. An unbooked pregnant woman presents to the labour ward with a small antepartum haemorrhage and abdominal pain at approximately 32 weeks gestation. How will you manage this case?

3. Discuss the management of pregnancy in a woman who has suffered from recurrent miscarriages and is diagnosed to have primary antiphospho-lipid syndrome.

4. What are the current controversies in management of toxoplasmosis in pregnancy?

5. The community midwife refers a primigravida at 26 weeks gestation as small for dates. Ultrasound reveals molar changes in the placenta. Discuss her further management.

## GYNAECOLOGY

1. Debate the options of management for a woman who has missed miscarriage at 10 weeks of pregnancy.

2. Discuss the controversy surrounding prophylactic oophorectomy.

3. How will you approach a 26-year-old woman who has been referred with recurrent vulvovaginal discharge over the past 2 years?

4. A 30-year-old nurse is referred by her GP because of a borderline smear. She gives a history of exposure to diethylstilbestrol *in utero*. What are the possible effects of this exposure and how will you counsel her?

5. You are presenting a proposal for the setting up of an early pregnancy assessment unit at your hospital. Discuss the pros and cons of such a unit.

# Index

abdominal incisions in gynaecological surgery, optimizing outcome 235
abdominal pain 126, 149
  during periods, clinical approach 208–9
abdominal wall defect in fetus 196
abortion 28
Abortion Act 29
abruptio placentae 72, 181
acid–base status 86
activated protein C resistance (APCR) 94
active management 17
acyclovir 64
adenomyosis 31
adhesions 144
adnexal torsion 169–70
adrenocorticotropic hormone 222
adriamycin 233
air embolism 158
alopecia 233
alpha thalassaemia 14
alphafetoprotein 196
Alzheimer's disease 189
amenorrhoea 39, 102, 126, 185–6
amniocentesis 90, 220
amnioinfusion 86
amniotic fluid 86, 162
  decompression 180
  embolism 158
amniotomy 176, 218
anaerobic vaginosis 154
anaesthesia 184
anaesthetic toxicity 158
aneuploidy, antenatal screening for 137
antenatal beds 72
antenatal care 154, 156
antibiotics 199, 201, 204, 234, 235
anticardiolipin antibody 94
anticholinergics 187
anticoagulants 235
anticonvulsants 89
anti-D 118–19, 126
antiemetics 222
antihistamine 114
antihypertensives 199
antiphospholipid (APL) antibodies 94
antiphospholipid (APL) syndrome 94

antiprostaglandins 21
anti-retroviral treatment 160
anti-thrombin III 76, 94
antiviral drugs 64
Apgar score 86, 178
artificial rupture of membranes (ARM) 197
ascites 13
aspirin 94, 208
atosiban 21, 22
avascular necrosis 204
Ayre's spatula 81
azathioprine 216

bacterial vaginosis 13, 18, 94, 201
behavioural therapy 187
beta agonists 21, 22
beta haemolytic streptococci 201
bilateral mastectomy 34
bilateral oophorectomy 34, 104, 189
bilateral pleural effusion 13, 14
bile acids 114
biophysical profile (BPP) 162
biopsy 164
Bird's occipito-posterior metal cup 134
Bishop's score 140, 218
bisphosphonates 77
bladder damage 204
bladder injury 182
bladder repair 182
bladder retraining 187
blood tests 158
blood transfusion 144
  patient's decision to decline 92–3
body mass index (BMI) 18
Bolam test 129
bowel injury at laparoscopy 106–7
brainstorming 5
BRCA1 or BRCA2 gene mutation 32, 33
breast cancer 27, 30, 32, 36, 189
breast self-examination 228
breastfeeding 160, 216
breech presentation 48–9
bromocriptine 185

cabergoline 186
caesarean section 25, 48, 64, 86, 87, 92, 134, 136, 140, 148, 156, 157, 159, 160, 178, 195, 201, 218, 224

caesarean section (*contd*)
  informed decision 224
  management 182
  prevention 176
  rising rate and steps to reduce it 44
  risks and benefits 224
  *see also* vaginal birth after caesarean section (VBAC)
calcium channel blockers 22
cancer 32
cancer treatment 167–8
carboplatin 233
cardiopulmonary resuscitation 158
cardiotocography (CTG) 44, 48, 86, 140, 176, 201
cataracts 189
cautery 235
cephalic presentation 140, 224
  informed decision 224
cephalosporins 50
cerebral haemorrhage 158
cervical cancer 151
cervical cerclage 95
cervical cytology 98
cervical glandular intraepithelial neoplasia (CGIN) 80
  examination 80
  follow-up cytology 81
  investigations 80
  management 80
cervical intraepithelial neoplasia (CIN) 98, 151
  conservative management 98–9
  grade III 229–30
  investigations 98
  natural history 98
  surgical management 98
cervical pathology 82
cervical priming 167
cervical smear screening 80, 151–2, 228–30
cervical squamous carcinoma 122
cervicitis 82
chemoprophylaxis 33
chickenpox 112
chlamydia screening 191–2
chlorpheniramine 114
chorioamnionitis 141, 181
chromosomal anomalies 14
chronic pelvic inflammatory disease 149
cisplatin 233
clam ileocystoplasty 187
clean intermittent self-catheterization (CISC) 187, 188
cleidotomy 70
clindamycin 201
clinical audits 174
clomiphene citrate 35, 124

clomiphene-resistant PCOS 210
$CO_2$ laser vaporization 165
coagulopathy 159
cocaine 154
Cochrane Collaboration 7–8
Cochrane Controlled Trials Register (CCTR) 8
Cochrane Database of Systematic Reviews (CDSR) 7
Cochrane Review Methodology Database (CRMD) 8
codeine 208
colon cancer 189
colpocleisis 130
colposcopy 98, 164, 229–30
combined abdominoperineal procedure 130–1
combined oral contraceptives 146, 179
complaints procedure 174
computer-assisted homography (CT) scan 122, 185
concurrent oophorectomy 60
Confidential Enquiry into Peri-operative Deaths (CEPOD) 184
congenital diaphragmatic hernia 66
  antenatal period 66
  delivery period 66
  postnatal period 67
congenital rubella syndrome 112
congenital varicella syndrome 46
consent 128
contraception 54, 78, 102, 128, 167, 217
  discontinuation 146
  documentation 55
  follow-up 55
cord platelet count 157
cord prolapse 148, 218
cordocentesis 14, 156
corticosteroids 180, 201, 216, 222
counselling 10, 33, 38, 39, 46, 48, 54, 60, 66, 79, 99, 128, 140, 160–1, 171–2, 182, 199, 216–17, 220
Crohn's disease 216–17
  antenatal 216
  delivery 216
  postpartum 216
  preconceptual 216
culdocentesis 100
Cushing's syndrome 166
cycle cancellation 171
cyclo-oxygenase 2 (COX-2) inhibitors 21
cyclophosphamide 233
cyproterone acetate 36, 166
cystic hygroma 14
cystodistension 187
cystoscopy 122
cytology 151
cytomegalovirus 112

D immunoglobulin 118–19
day assessment unit 72
  advantages 72
  disadvantages 72–3
debulking surgery 212
deep vein thrombosis (DVT) 76, 78, 179, 184
delivery
  Crohn's disease 216
  drug addiction 154
  ITP 156
delivery options in prolonged second stage labour 134
delivery suite, risk management 174
Depo-Provera 146
detrusor instability 204
  management options 187–8
diabetes mellitus 68, 178, 218
  diagnostic test 68
  history 68
  proposed model 69
  risk factors 68
  screening tests 68
  uncontrolled 72
diagnosis 9, 19
Dianette 36
diathermy 210
dietary restriction 178
differential diagnoses 158
dinitrochlorobenzene 164
disseminated intravascular coagulation (DIC) 138
DNA amplification tests 191
Doppler studies 42, 154, 162, 201
  cons 42
  pros 42
  uses 42
Down's syndrome 90–1, 137, 220
  recurrence risk 91
drug addiction 154
dRVVT 94
ductal constriction 180
ductus arteriosus, premature closure 180
dysfunctional uterine bleeding (DUB) 30
dyskaryosis 98, 229
  protocol for management 229
dysmenorrhoea 31, 39, 208
dyspareunia 149

ectopic pregnancy 126, 167–71, 191
endocervical brush 81
endometrial ablation 27, 38
endometrial biopsy 58
endometrial cancer 36, 189
endometrial hyperplasia 30, 31
endometriosis 144, 149, 167

endoscopic ligation 220
enterocoele 130
epidural analgesia 110, 156
epidural cannula 178
epilepsy 88–9
episiotomy 70, 195
epithelial ovarian cancer
  morbidity associated with chemotherapy 233–4
  surgery in 212–13
erythroblastosis fetalis 118–19
  reasons for decrease in incidence 118
  reasons for persistence 118
essay answers
  basic steps 4–7
  structuring 9–10
evidence-based medicine 7
expectant management 17, 90
external cephalic version (ECV) 48, 218–19
extraction of posterior arm 70
extraperitonization 182

factor V Leiden deficiency 76, 78
factor XIII 94
fallopioscopy 100–1
female sterilization 103, 147
  litigation in relation to 128
  medicolegal issues 128–9
fenamates 208
Fenton's operation 195
fertility 146, 228
fertility-preserving surgery 122
fetal abnormalities 162
fetal blood sampling 86, 90
fetal congenital heart disease 162
fetal death 13, 16
  twin pregnancy 138–9
fetal growth abnormalities 162
fetal growth restriction 72
fetal heart rate (FHR) monitoring 86–7
fetal intracranial haemorrhage 156
fetal lung maturation 201
fetal macrosomia 162
fetal monitoring 25, 86, 176, 197
fetal morbidity and mortality 48
fetal platelet count 156
fetal scalp blood sampling (FBS) 86, 176
fetal scalp monitoring 156
fetomaternal haemorrhage (FMH) 118
fibroids 31, 82, 167
flavoxate 187
fluid restriction 187
5-fluorouracil 164
folic acid 216
food-borne infections 113
forceps delivery 70–1, 134, 194

FSH 102
functional bowel disorders 149

galactorrhoea 185
gamete intrafallopian transfer (GIFT) 124
*Gardnerella vaginalis* 18
gas hydrotubation 100
gastrointestinal disturbance 122
genetic counselling 91
genetic screening 33
genitourinary anomalies 14
genuine stress incontinence 204
glucose tolerance test (GTT) 68–9, 95
gonadotrophin releasing hormone (GnRH) 38, 104
gonadotrophins 36, 124, 210
graft rejection 199
grand mal epilepsy 88–9

Haemaccel 92
haematinics 92
haematological disorders 14
haematoma 178
haemoglobin 92
haemorrhage 72, 92, 130
Hasson technique 106
healthy lifestyle 77, 124, 189
heparin 83–4, 94, 159, 179, 231
   side effects 84
hepatitis B 154
hepatitis C 154
hepatorenal failure 223
herpes
   antenatal treatment 64
   postnatal care 64–5
   treatment 64
heterotopic pregnancy 126, 171
high-dose combined oral contraceptive pill (pc4) 54
hirsutism 27, 35, 36, 166
   history and examination 166
   investigations 166
   treatment 166
histopathology 164
HIV screening 160–1
HIV test 154
hormone replacement therapy (HRT) 31, 58, 60, 76–7, 102, 189, 228
human papillomavirus (HPV) DNA 151–2
human papillomavirus (HPV) test 151–2
hydrocephalus 162
hydronephrosis 162
hyperemesis gravidarum 72
   investigations 222–3
   management 222–3
   potential complications 222–3
hyperinsulinaemia 35, 36

hyperprolactinaemia 185
hypofibrinogenaemia 16
hypophysectomy 166
hypothyroidism 185
hysterectomy 60, 92, 189
   laparoscopy in 144
   potential urological consequences 204–5
hysterosalpingo-contrast-sonography (HyCoSy) 100
hysterosalpingogram (HSG) 100
hysteroscopy 95

idiopathic polyhydramnios 180–1
ileostomy 216–17
imipramine 187
immune thrombocytopoenic purpura (ITP) 156–7
immunosuppressants 199
implant removal 146
incident forms 174
incisional hernia 235
indomethacin 21, 180, 201
induction of labour (IOL) 116–17, 181, 201
   complications 116
   informed decision 116–17
   large baby 135
   vs. conservative management 140
infection
   in pregnancy 112–13
   prevention 178
infertility 122, 124–5, 191, 210
   treatment 35
inotropes 158
in-patient hysteroscopy 58
interferon 164
intermenstrual bleeding 122
Internet 8–9
intracardiac potassium chloride 90
intracytoplasmic sperm injection (ICSI) 61, 125, 171
   advantages 61
   candidates 61–2
   potential disadvantages 61
intrahepatic cholestasis of pregnancy (ICP) 114–15
   delivery/surgical management 115
   investigations 114
   medical treatment 114
   postnatal care 115
   prognosis 114
   supportive management 114
intrapartum death 24
intrapartum electronic fetal monitoring 13, 24
intrapartum fetal hypoxia 197
intrauterine contraceptive device (IUCD) 146
   lost threads 206
   refitting 206

removal 206
replacement 228
surgical removal 206
intrauterine death 16
intrauterine device (IUD) 54, 102
intrauterine growth restriction (IUGR) 148, 199
intrauterine infections 14
intrauterine insemination 124
intravenous crystalloid 92
intravenous immunoglobulin (IVIG) 156
intravenous urogram 148
in vitro fertilization (IVF) 61, 125, 171–2, 220
irritable bowel syndrome adhesions 149

Jehovah's Witness 92

karyotyping 90
Kielland's forceps 134
Kleihauer test 118

labour, slow progress in active phase of first stage 197–8
labour ward guidelines 176
labour ward protocols 174, 179
lamotrigine 88
laparoscopic chromopertubation 100
laparoscopic ovarian diathermy (LOD) 210–11
laparoscopic sacrocolpopexy 131
laparoscopic salpingotomy 126
laparoscopy 95, 124, 126, 128, 150, 169–70, 209, 211
bowel injury 106–7
in hysterectomy 144
laparotomy 126, 231
large baby 135–6
clinical examination 135
induction of labour 135
investigations 135
verification of suspicion 135
large loop excision of transformation zone (LLETZ) 80, 98
Le Fort's operation 130
leiomyoma 167
leukaemia 234
levonorgestrel intrauterine system (LNG-IUS) 27, 30, 31, 54, 102, 146
listeriosis 113
litigation in relation to female sterilization 128
liver function tests 95, 114
lower segment caesarean section (LSCS) 134, 156, 181
luteinizing hormone (LH) 35
lymph nodes 122

macroadenoma 185
McRobert's manoeuvre 70

macroprolactinomas 185–6
macrosomia 178
magnesium sulphate 21, 22
magnetic resonance imaging (MRI) 122, 138, 150, 185
malignancy 164
malpresentation 148
mammogram 33
management 9
maternal blood pressure 178
maternal blood tests 14
maternal platelet count 157
maternal serology 156
maternal serum alpha fetoprotein 88
meconium 86
medicolegal issues in female sterilization 128–9
MEDLINE 7, 8
medroxyprogesterone acetate 36, 102
mefenamic acid 208
menopause 60, 76
menorrhagia 27, 31, 38, 60, 82, 102, 228
menstrual periods 27, 35
menstruation 102
methylene blue test 100
metronidazole 201, 216
microadenoma 185
midfollicular LH/FSH 94
midtrimester bleeding 72
mifepristone 29, 167–8
Mirena intrauterine system 228
miscarriage 18, 19, 94–5, 148, 162, 210, 216
misoprostol 28
mock examinations 237
molar pregnancy 56
investigations 56
medical treatment 56
supportive management 56
surgical treatment 56
multidisciplinary care 158
multiple pregnancy 171–2, 210
mutation testing 32
myelosuppression 234
myocardial infarction 158

nausea 222
neonatal cranial ultrasound 138
neonatal death 14
neonatal infection 141
nephrectomy 51
nephrotoxic agents 233
neuromodulation 187
nevirapine 160
nifedipine 21, 201
non-immune hydrops fetalis (NIFH) 14, 15
norethisterone enanthate 102

Norplant 146
nuchal fold translucency (NFT) 137

obesity in pregnancy 178–9
oligohydramnios 162
occipito-anterior position 134
oestrogen pills 89
oestrogen therapy 189
oligomenorrhoea 31
omphalocele 196
oophorectomy 60
opiates 154
osteoporosis 76, 189
out-patient endometrial biopsy 58
out-patient saline hysterography 58–9
out-patient sonohysteroscopy 58–9
ovarian cancer 27, 32, 60
ovarian conservation 122
ovarian failure 122
ovarian hyperstimulation 171, 210
ovarian hyperstimulation syndrome (OHSS) 231
    history and examination 231
    investigations 231
    presentation and management 231
    treatment 231
ovarian stimulation protocol 124
ovaries, removal 60
ovulation induction 124
oxybutynin 187
oxygenation 158
oxytocics 92, 110
oxytocin 21, 22, 116, 140, 176, 197, 198

paclitaxel 233
pain relief 154
palliative surgery 213
Palmer's test 106
parental karyotyping 94
parenteral nutrition 223
parvovirus B19 112
pelvic floor, potential injuries 194
pelvic infection 171
pelvic inflammatory disease (PID) 169–70, 191
pelvic lymphadenectomy 122
pelvic pain 149, 169–70, 191
    examination 149
    history 149
    investigations 149
pelvic ultrasound scanning 94, 150
penicillin 50, 201
periodontal disease 189
perioperative morbidity and mortality in gynaeco-
    logical surgery 184–5
periovarian adhesions 211
PGE2 116

phenytoin sodium 88
pituitary imaging 185
placenta praevia 48, 72, 218
placental adherence 148
planning the answer 6
platelet transfusion 157
polycystic ovarian syndrome (PCOS) 210–11
polycystic ovaries 35, 36, 94, 185, 210
polyhydramnios 66, 135, 162, 180–1, 218
postcoital bleeding 122
postmature pregnancy 86
postmortem 14
postnatal care 155, 157
post-pill amenorrhoea 146
potassium chloride 126, 220
practice questions 239–43
pregnancy
    clinical diagnosis 178
    twin 138–9, 162, 220
    see also specific aspects
pregnancy-associated placental protein (PAPPA)
    137
pregnancy-induced hypertension 72, 199
pregnancy test 128, 185
premature menopause 105
premature rupture of membranes 72
premenstrual syndrome (PMS) 31, 39, 60, 104–5
    history 104
    hormonal treatment 104
    investigation 104
    medical (non-hormonal) treatment 104
    supportive treatment 104
    surgical treatment 104
prepregnancy clinic 94–5
preterm delivery 199
    twin pregnancy 139
preterm labour 148, 162, 180, 181, 210
preterm premature rupture of membranes
    (PPROM) 181, 201
progesterone-only pill 54, 89, 102, 146
progestogens 103, 189
prolactin 185
propantheline bromide 187
propiverine hydrochloride 187
prostaglandin 140
prostaglandin synthetase inhibitors 180
proteins C and S 76, 94
pruritus 114
Pseudomonas 234
psychosexual counselling 165
pulmonary embolism 158
pulmonary malformations 14
pyelonephritis 50
    follow-up 50
    investigations 50

medical treatment 50
supportive management 50
surgical treatment 51
pyonephrosis 51
pyridoxine 222

radical hysterectomy 122
radical trachelectomy 122
radiotherapy 122
raloxifene 189
recanalization 128
recurrent miscarriage 18, 19
investigations 94
renal function tests 95
renal tract abnormalities 148
renal transplantation 199
respiratory distress syndrome (RDS) 21, 138
retroperitoneal lymphadenectomy 122
Rhesus immunization 118
risk analysis 174
risk assessment 9
risk control 174
risk identification 174
ritodrine 201
rotational forceps 134
RU 486 167
rubella 112

sacrocolpopexy 130
sacrospinous ligament fixation 130
salpingectomy 126
salpingo-oophorectomy 60
salpingotomy 126
SATFA (Support Around Termination for Fetal Abnormality) 90–1
scalp oedema 13, 14
screening 10
second-look laparoscopy or laparotomy 213
selective salpingography 100–1
selective screening 19
selective termination (ST) 220
septic shock 158
serial growth scans 154
serum screening 137
sexually transmitted infection 191
short-term voiding disorders 204
shoulder dystocia 70–1, 136, 179
sling operation 130
spironolactone 166
spontaneous rupture of membranes 86–7, 140, 201, 218
squamous carcinoma of cervix 122
staging laparotomy 212
steroids 114, 138, 156, 199
stillbirth 14, 162

Strassman's prodedure 148
subarachnoid haemorrhage 158
subtotal abdominal hysterectomy 82
potential benefits 82
potential disadvantages 82
suction curettage 56
sulphasalazine 216
superovulation 124
suprapubic catheterization 182
suprasellar extension 185
sutures 235
Swan-Ganz catheter 158
symphysiofundal height 135
symphysiotomy 70

tamoxifen 30–2
teratogenic effects 199
teratogenic infectious exposure 14
terfenadine 114
termination of pregnancy (TOP) 27–9, 90, 137, 167–8, 196, 223, 231
termination of twin pregnancy 220
therapeutic thoracentesis 66
thiamine 222
third generation progestogen 78
thrombocytopoenia 84, 233
thromboembolic deterrent stockings 84
thromboembolism 189
thrombophilia 76, 78, 94
thromboprophylaxis 231
thyroid enlargement 185
thyroid function tests 95
tibolone 77, 189
tocolytics 13, 21, 201
Tomkin's procedure 148
TORCH screen 95
toxoplasmosis 113
transdermal therapy 76
transvaginal ultrasound scan 58, 126
trial of labour 110
tricuspid regurgitation 180
trisomy 21 90
tubal ligation 147
tubal patency in infertility 100–1
tubo-ovarian abscess 169
twin pregnancy 138–9, 162, 220
preterm delivery 139

ultrasonography 58
ultrasound scanning 14, 92, 135, 148, 154, 162, 180, 196, 208
unipolar diathermy 220
unstable lie 72, 218–19
history and examination 218
investigations 218

unstable lie (*contd*)
  management 218–19
ureteric damage 204–5
urinary tract infection 182, 199, 204
urogenital anomalies 95
ursodeoxycholic acid 114
uterine hypotonia 176
uterine malformation 148
uterine rupture 148
uterosacral ligaments 130

vaginal birth after caesarean section (VBAC) 110–11
  management issues 110
  risks and benefits 110
vaginal bleeding 56, 58
vaginal delivery
  potential harmful effects 194–5
  trial 48–9
vaginal discharge 38
vaginal stenosis 122
vaginal vault prolapse 130–1
varicella 46
  counselling 46
  history 46
  investigations 46
vasectomy 103, 147
venous thromboembolism following surgery 83–4
  high-risk patients 83
  moderate risk factors 83

preoperative assessment 83
ventilation 158
ventouse delivery 134, 194
vertical transmission 160
vitamin K 88, 114
vitamin suppliements 222
vomiting 222
vulval herpetic lesions 64
vulvar epithelia neoplasia (VIN) 164–5
  investigations 164
  natural history 164
  treatment 164–5

warfarin 76
Wernick's encephalopathy 222
Wood's corkscrew manoeuvre 70
World Wide Web 7
wound dehiscence 235
wound drains 235
wound haematoma 235
wound infection 235

Y chromosome 171
York Database of Abstracts of Reviews of Effectiveness (DARE) 8

Zacharin's procedure 130–1
Zavanelli's manoeuvre 70
zidovudine 160
zoster immume globulin (ZIG) 46